An introduction to psycho-oncology

T0175861

One in three of us will develop cancer. It is extremely common and in many situations a truly frightening disease, yet for too long the psychological aspects have been ignored. In *An Introduction to Psycho-Oncology* Professor Patrice Guex has put together a comprehensive and up-to-date guide, reviewing current thinking on the subject of a possible psychosomatic aetiology of cancer, on the emotional and psychological reactions that it provokes, and on the treatments available.

Illustrated with eleven case histories, the book deals in a clear and simple manner with the reactions of cancer patients to their illness. It touches on every aspect of cancer care, including pain relief, psycho-pharmacology, and complementary medicine, and gives special attention to the needs of terminal patients and their carers. Professor Guex looks at the cancer patient as a whole person and brings to his or her support every means available to enhance the quality of life, including the concept of self-help and the transfer of power from the professional to the client.

Primarily intended for all doctors, nurses and professionals working with cancer patients, *An Introduction to Psycho-Oncology* will also be helpful to leaders of cancer support groups and to people who are themselves living with cancer.

Patrice Guex is Associate Professor in the Department of Adult Psychology at the University of Lausanne, Switzerland, and Medical Director of the Division of Psycho-Social Medicine at the Centre Hospitalier Universitaire Vaudois, Lausanne.
Heather Goodare experienced cancer in 1986 and, finding there was little psychological support available for cancer patients, decided to train as a counsellor. She now practises privately, and is active in voluntary work with cancer self-help organizations.

An introduction to psycho-oncology

Patrice Guex

Translated by Heather Goodare

Foreword by Karol Sikora

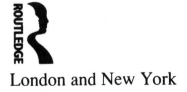

London and New York

The original French edition of this book was published in
1989, under the title *Psychologie et cancer, manuel de psycho-
oncologie*, by Editions Payot Lausanne.

© 1989 Editions Payot Lausanne

First English (revised) edition published in 1994
by Routledge
11 New Fetter Lane, London EC4P 4EE

Simultaneously published in the USA and Canada
by Routledge
29 West 35th Street, New York, NY 10001

© 1994 Heather Goodare and Patrice Guex for the English
translation; Foreword: Karol Sikora

Typeset in 10/12pt Times by
Ponting–Green Publishing Services, Chesham, Bucks

British Library Cataloguing in Publication Data
A catalogue record for this book is available from the British Library.

Library of Congress Cataloging in Publication Data
Guex, Patrice.
    [Psychologie et cancer. English]
    An introduction to psycho-oncology/Patrice Guex; translated by
    Heather Goodare; foreword by Karl Sikora.
        p.cm.
    Includes bibliographical references and index.
    1. Cancer–Psychological aspects.
    2. Cancer–Psychosomatic aspects.
    I. Title   II. Title: Introduction to psychooncology.
    [DNLM: 1. Neoplasms–psychology.   QZ 200 G939p 1993a]
    RC262.99'4'0019–dc20
    DNLM/DLC
    for Library of Congress   93–15029
                                                                    CIP

ISBN 0–415–06435–x (hbk)
ISBN 0–415–06436–8 (pbk)

Contents

Tables

Foreword

One in three of us will develop cancer. It is extremely common and in many situations a truly frightening disease. Nowhere in medicine is there such interaction between the holistic trinity of body, mind, and spirit. Over the last decade there has been a new wave of honesty in the way in which health-care professionals communicate with cancer patients. People now know they have cancer; they understand the treatment options and their side-effects, and the likely chances of success. This new frankness brings with it new stresses for patients and their carers as well as for health-care professionals. For too long the psychological aspects of cancer have been ignored. Now, at last, they are receiving intense scrutiny as we strive to improve the total package of cancer care that we provide.

There are few comprehensive source-books from which to start. Here Professor Guex, a Lausanne psychiatrist with considerable experience in the problems facing cancer patients, has put together an excellent and up-to-date primer. Clearly translated by Heather Goodare – a cancer patient herself – it captures the essence of the subject, transcending with ease any language and cultural barriers.

It first considers the controversial relationship of psychological factors in the causation of cancer and the various psychobiological models that have been developed. The vexed question of the 'cancer personality' is perhaps one of the most enigmatic problems that causes heated discussion. The way in which patients adapt to illness – with denial, anger, acceptance, and helplessness – and the changes in the quality of life are outlined. There then follows a series of chapters on the interaction between the patient and the provision of conventional therapies: surgery, radiotherapy, and chemotherapy. The sections on pain control and the psychopharmacology of cancer provide useful prescribing information for the physician.

The problems of those providing care in cancer treatment centres often result in stress and interpersonal difficulties. This can lead to potentially disastrous power games, which in turn can lead to an almost complete communication breakdown, much to the patients' disadvantage. The causes of these changes are analysed and the benefits of the multidisciplinary team as a load-sharing device to defuse conflict are highlighted. Complementary and indeed alternative therapies are discussed, together with the concept of self-help and the transfer of power from professional to client.

The book is easy to read and flows well. It is studded with useful examples from Professor Guex's personal experience. The bibliography provides a comprehensive entrée into the literature. I would commend it to all who deal with cancer patients, whatever their professional background. There is no doubt that it will help in understanding the most difficult and challenging aspect of caring for cancer – dealing with the patient's mind. If there is one take-home message for all of us, it is Professor Guex's invocation to 'listen to the patient'.

Karol Sikora
Professor of Clinical Oncology,
Royal Postgraduate Medical School,
Hammersmith Hospital, London

Preface to the revised edition

The current fashion in psychosocial oncology in the Anglo-Saxon world is to evaluate the psycho-emotional problems of the cancer patient in a scientifically rigorous manner. I am therefore particularly amused to find that this little book, originally written for French and Italian readers, which is concerned with daily life, with emotions, with clinical experience, and so with the qualitative, not to say anecdotal, should have found its own way, without my help, as far as England.

Perhaps this should not surprise me, because in my clinical work with cancer patients I hear so many unexpected stories, and I am particularly inclined to favour their 'narrative reconstructions', their valuation of their existential experience, when they lose hope and are completely absorbed by their illness, the problems which it brings, and the loss of meaning in their lives. I take this opportunity to thank my patients (or their relatives) for permission to quote their case histories in this book, though details that might identify them have been removed.

So this manual of psycho-oncology, whose history I had imagined was finished, now has an unexpected new lease of life, thanks to the tenacity and enterprise of Heather Goodare, who has not only produced an excellent translation but also undertaken its promotion.

I am particularly grateful to her because, with the strength gained from her own experience of life and from her training as a counsellor, she has been able to put her finger on many omissions and doubtful points, which we have reconsidered together. She has also made a valuable contribution to the revision of the chapter on complementary medicine, which perhaps took insufficient account of the available adjuvant therapies that now contribute to holistic care and help to give patients good socio-affective relationships and the best possible quality of life.

She has also assured me that in Great Britain and the United States there is still room for deep reflection on the needs of patients and the carer–client relationship, alongside scientific approaches and epidemiological studies. Her message is thus one of hope and of complementarity.

Patrice Guex
Associate Professor
Department of Adult Psychiatry, University of Lausanne
Medical Director
Department of Psycho-Social Medicine,
Centre Universitaire Hospitalier Vaudois, Lausanne

Translator's note

The story of how I came upon this book by chance in the course of a cycling tour of Brittany, and went on to translate it, is an apt illustration of a cancer patient's search for meaning: one of the themes touched on by the author.

In preparing this new edition for English-speaking readers, I have been very grateful for helpful comments from the following: Dr Ann Johnson, Hon. Consultant Surgical Oncologist, Breast Study Centre, Mount Vernon Hospital; Dr David Julier, Consultant Psychiatrist, Littlemore Hospital, Oxford; Dr Michael Crowe, Consultant Psychiatrist, The Maudsley Hospital; Dr James Lurie, Clinical Professor of Psychiatry, University of Washington; Dr Jane Foster; Dr Gillian O'Donnell; John Foster, Educational Psychologist; Mitchell Noon, Specialist in Health Psychology, University of Sussex; Christopher Greatorex, Psychotherapist; May Bullen, Macmillan Support Nurse, Crawley Hospital; Ashley Adsett, Oncology Counsellor, Royal Sussex County Hospital, Brighton; and Philip Tyler, Counsellor. I am also grateful to my husband, Kenneth Goodare, for his patience and support during the course of the work, and for his contributions to early drafts.

Finally, Professor Karol Sikora has been a constant source of encouragement, and the author himself, an inspiration. However, none of these people is in any way accountable for any remaining inaccuracies or infelicities in the translation, which are entirely my responsibility.

The question of gender deserves mention. In French, grammatical gender does not necessarily coincide with sex (for example, a person is always *une personne*, which of course includes the male as well as the female). In English in order to be politically correct we resort to clumsy devices such as 'him/her' or refer to people alternately as male and female, which can give rise to awkwardness and ambiguity. I have preferred to use the male gender throughout where the female is also intended, except for cases where the person referred to is invariably female. I should like to assure readers that I am as good a feminist as anyone.

This translation is dedicated to the memory of Shirley Toms, who fought cancer bravely and whose story illustrates so many of the themes in this book.

Heather Goodare
Horsham, West Sussex

Introduction

Recent advances in oncology have made possible an improvement in the survival rates of patients. We may now expect long-term remissions, and cures, but these require sustained effort and sacrifices on the part of patients and their families.

Health professionals, for their part, are faced with the problems of much more complex, multifaceted treatments, which may be described in a rather broad manner in terms of the 'global approach to the patient'. But we must be aware above all of the human and existential dimensions of the disease. We can no longer ignore the psychological, psychosocial, and behavioural aspects of cancer. It must be possible to take into consideration pain, anxiety, depression, the impairment of cognitive functions, and the quality of life, both during and after treatment. Health-care teams can no longer allow themselves to wait until the patient becomes 'symptomatic' or until he manifests his disorder before looking at the possibility of providing appropriate support. For every situation, they now have the duty to assess the needs of the patient and his relatives, at each stage of the disease and of the treatments. That implies, of course, the planning of interventions, a co-ordination of services, and an ongoing sustained dialogue between the various people engaged in the task.

This therapeutic partnership (*médecine d'accompagnement*) integrates not only the most recent scientific discoveries but also the various means of support which patients need to understand their disease and their treatment, and to adapt to it.

The present *Introduction to Psycho-Oncology* does not claim to be in any sense exhaustive. Even if it did, this objective would be impossible to achieve. It is in fact unwise to promote only one way of working in a field where personal preparation, sensitivity, and motivation play such an essential part. The different chapters of this book offer an overview of the important topics which must be considered. Certain themes have not been touched on, notably that of children with cancer. This is a speciality in itself, which requires a long training and which I leave to other, more competent colleagues.

If I had to sum up the hours I have spent with cancer patients, I would venture to do it in the following way: there are certain precise facts which one must know and which are useful. The most important one, however, is given to us by the patient himself. He shares with us a dramatic moment, of extreme emotional intensity. To train oneself in 'psycho-oncology' is perhaps to explore one's own limits, and above all to be prepared to listen to patients and to comprehend their distress, before, possibly, knowing what to do to help them.

Chapter 1

Psychosomatics and cancer

PSYCHOSOMATICS

Psychosomatic research in the study of cancer has existed for a long time. Many authors have tried to establish links between psychological problems and the onset of cancer. They have primarily engaged in retrospective studies, starting with isolated cases where there was a striking correlation between emotional traumas and the appearance of tumours after a certain delay (Abse 1964; Abse *et al.* 1973; Bahnson and Bahnson 1964; Bahnson 1969, 1975; Baltrusch 1956, 1975; Booth 1969). Longitudinal prospective studies, with more elaborate methodology, are rare; in broad outline, they share the conclusions of the former studies (Thomas and Greenstreet 1973; Thomas and Duszynski 1974; Greer and Morris 1975; Fox 1978; Greer *et al.* 1979). In his work of synthesis, Bammer (1981) has reviewed about two hundred works.

A central observation seems to run unanimously through all these publications: the experience, in the course of patients' lives, of separation, emotional upheavals (for example, divorce), or very painful bereavements, often cumulative, and without the possibility of working through them in a favourable environment (LeShan 1963).

Galen, in the second century AD, thought that melancholic women were predisposed to breast cancer. This theme was taken up again in the eighteenth century by Gendron (1701), who found that his patients who suffered from depression and anxiety were more subject to cancer. Guy (1759) added a little more detail by observing that nervous and hysterical women developed cancer after existential traumas and bereavements.

In the nineteenth century, it was asserted that reverses of fortune, bad socio-economic conditions and 'mental misery' are at the source of carcinomas (Walshe 1846). In 1900, there was renewed insistence on the influence of emotional losses, bereavement, and melancholy. Evans, in 1926, was the first to formulate the basis for oncological psychodynamics, after having studied the material obtained in the course of a hundred psychotherapeutic treatments.

The losses in question can go back to early childhood and be reactivated by the events of adult life, sometimes several years before the appearance of the first symptoms of the disease (Wirsching *et al.* 1982). 'Loss' and 'lack' seem to underlie the predisposition to cancer; to surmount this loss, the patient appears to have denied suffering so as to hyperadapt to reality, to the detriment of his emotional life. This would allow one to consider it as a psycho-somatic construct, characterized by a rigid mental attitude, difficulty in expressing emotions, and a restricted capacity for forming relation-ships (Marty and M'Uzan 1963; Fain 1966). The doctor, in fact, is often faced with patients who present a virgin and uneventful psychological case history, a rather disquieting lack of capacity for depression, and with whom a dialogue, apart from small talk, is very difficult to engage in because of problems in making contact. These difficulties are not immediately noticeable, for everything seems to be working out for the best, but they appear as soon as one can test the possibility of a genuine encounter (Schneider 1969b). Certain authors have observed that their patients have oral fixations, which lead to their forming asymmetrical relationships of dependence on others, where altruism and the search for harmony are pursued to the detriment of their own interests. Attachment to others is a way of reassuring oneself and of fighting depression. Any failure in this system, appearing in adult life, inevitably gives rise to the reopening of early wounds. The consequence of this is a kind of psychosomatic regression, with emotional isolation, which seems to provide fertile soil for the growth of cancer (Rusch 1944; Fisher 1967; Vaillant 1977; Greenberg and Dattore 1981).

Thomas and Duszynski (1974) attempted to validate such observa-tions by putting in hand a prospective study of a group of students at an American university. Those who were to develop cancer later were characterized by inability to express feelings, and they de-scribed their parents as cold and distant: for them, the repression and denial of affects seem to be bad prognostic factors. For Reznikoff (1955; Reznikoff and Martin 1957), women attacked by breast cancer are maladapted psychosexually and have been dominated by their mothers. LeShan (LeShan and Worthington 1956a; LeShan 1966), who studied 500 cancer patients over twelve years, discovered that three-quarters of them had had a traumatic experience, symbolic or actual, in childhood. Studying a group of breast cancer patients, Schmale and Iker (1964, 1966) noted that the longer the 'lagtime' before consultation, the more patients had recourse to denial, felt powerless to modify the course of their lives, and were socially isolated. They found a significant correlation between difficulty in communication and the development of tumours.

In taking as a base the psychological characteristics of cancer patients, Abse (1964) was able to determine, before any histological result, that 31 patients probably had lung cancer of the 59 who had to undergo a thoracotomy. Greer and Morris (1975) did the same, successfully predicting the result of breast lump biopsies on the basis of a psychological questionnaire. They described how the rate of malignancy was inversely proportional to the capacity to express aggression. Schonfield (1975), for his part, was less successful, in that he only managed to predict 27 cancerous lesions out of 112 biopsies, and he reckons that there is no correlation between malignancy and recent stressful event.

More generally, it has been noted that many behavioural factors have been associated with the onset of cancer. These factors seem to operate by way of several routes (Levy 1985), and we refer later to various cancer-related immunological processes. A large number of studies implicate several quite different types of psychosocial variables as predictors of cancer outcome (see Fox 1978 for a critical review). In the next section we see how a constellation of traits and coping styles may contribute to the 'cancer-prone personality'.

THE PSYCHODYNAMIC APPROACH

The 'cancer personality' has been graphically described by several authors, including Bahnson (1980).

Some patients have bad memories of their childhood, with the impression of having lacked affection, and above all of never having been able to express needs and feelings in the face of cold and distant parents. In such a context, to express one's resentments exposes one (in reality, or at least in one's imagination) to the threat of desertion and break-up. Apparently, the only way of keeping a protective framework is to compel affection, by exercising a strict control over oneself (so being precociously reasonable), and by subjecting oneself rigidly to social norms (that is to say, to begin with, to the supposed rules of one's parents).

Such a child can only maintain a harmonious relationship with his parents at the cost of great effort, in prematurely taking on too-heavy tasks, which goes together with a considerable feeling of inadequacy. This is one of the basic mechanisms of dependency. In adolescence, liberation is perceived as a too-painful deprivation, which one later tries to overcome by establishing bonds with an idealized object or by engaging with all one's energy in an intense activity (producing conflict between the ideal of the ego and reality). A new affective trauma in adulthood, if it is superimposed on such a history, can only be devastating. The individual, having learnt to be wary of his parents and to control his hostility towards them, transfers these feelings to his partner. When there is a break-up, the despair of infancy, up till now well camouflaged, springs up, reactivating all the old wounds.

Bereavement or divorce may precede the onset of cancer by several years. The patient, who has already more or less survived severe psychological difficulties since adolescence, is not equipped to cope with this new attack. He turns in on himself and becomes isolated from other people. This break-up involves a psychological regression to old ways of coping. Instead of expressing his suffering, his helplessness, his sadness, or his tragedy, the patient represses his emotions, as he learnt to do when younger. He tries to overcome everything stoically, head held high, and relying henceforth on his own strength alone. Thus pathological relationships are exacerbated, and the individual expects no help from others. He will put people off the track by appearing pleasant and adaptable. The cancer would thus appear as a sort of solution, a response to all expectations. Psychosomatic regression makes the body sick, but at the same time it gives one permission to have the right to say at last 'I suffer', to ask for help, perfectly justified this time, and at the same time to set limits. In fact, being ill also means not being able to respond to what one imagines to be the excessive expectations of others. It is also a way of saying: 'I am incapable of telling you what I want, but since you can't guess my needs, I will destroy myself.'

This psychodynamic model establishes a link between repeated emotional stress and cancer. One could say that we are dealing with people who have developed a double life, or a double self, or else a fundamental ambivalence, with on the one hand a definition of self well adapted to reality and to others, and on the other, deeply buried,

Table 1.1 The at-risk personality (after Bammer 1981)

1   Courtesy and cordiality
2   Submission to authority
3   Submission to social norms
4   Ready neglect of one's own feelings, and behaviour according to the general expectation of others
5   Sense of responsibility, conscientiousness, and zeal
6   Religiosity
7   Altruism and sense of sacrifice
8   Inhibition of aggressive feelings
9   Guilt, readiness to be self-critical, feeling of inferiority, depressive tendency

a 'phantom ego', which feels isolated, unloved, hurt, and often empty (Table 1.1).

THE SYSTEMIC APPROACH

We have seen that impassivity, rigidity of behaviour, struggle against depressive tendencies, and loneliness may result from affects that were inhibited during childhood; these are the mechanisms which are called 'repression' or denial and which may be secondary to the threats (supposed or actual) hanging over the unity of the family of origin (Kissen 1963; Bahnson and Bahnson 1964; Henderson 1966; Derogatis *et al.* 1979a). In this type of family, where mutual isolation and distancing are the rule, a certain precocious individuation is necessary, for the child can neither say who he is nor share his experiences with his relatives. It is in such conditions that, often, the repression of these negative feelings (sadness, anger, or jealousy) and the inhibition of desires appear in order to 'protect the family equilibrium': one has the impression that in such systems the emphasis is not on social opening-out, adaptation, and blossoming, but rather on self-mastery and control. Thus the future patient has made a habit of relying only on his own strength, and he expects no extra help from his family circle. It is precisely when he finally realizes that he is alone that he will fall ill. Certain studies (Greene 1966, Schmale and Iker 1966) seem to indicate that the passage of the family through an important stage of the life cycle – the emancipation of the children, for example – may also engender illness: breast cancer in the mother, or else leukaemia, Hodgkin's disease, or testicular cancer in the young (according to Minuchin's 1974 model of families with psychosomatic transactions). This would seem to be a decisive moment for activating a latent biological process. One could nevertheless doubt whether this scenario is specific to cancer and wonder if one has here enough elements to speak rather of a general tendency to illness than of a particular type of ailment. Indeed, according to certain authors (Hinkle *et al.* 1958; Greenberg and Dattore 1981), the patients who have the most risk factors do not inevitably develop cancers rather than other types of illness (cardiovascular for example), nor do they develop one type of cancer rather than another.

In conclusion, and with reference to the contextual theories of Boszormenyi-Nagy and Spark (1973), one could say that this type of cancer patient has had a career as a 'parentified child', preferring family stability to his own processes of individuation, in the face of unreceptive parents who offer few rewards. If the balance of 'debits and credits' is too unfavourable to the person who has followed such an itinerary, he will perhaps 'gain' this 'right to destroy', which is the source of many behavioural disorders and psychiatric problems. Further, depending on the degree of inability of the family to change, one could imagine that the patient turns this 'right to destroy' against himself, and that then the cancerous illness would correspond well with that 'narcissistic' regression described by other authors (Bahnson 1980).

BIOPSYCHOSOCIAL PERSPECTIVES

Some research suggests that behaviour, life-style, social environment, and stress play a part in the onset of cancer. It is in all probability the endocrine and immunological mechanisms which make the link between the context, the individual, and his organic carcinogenic determinants. The biopsychosocial model (Engel 1977) and general systems theory (von Bertalanffy 1964) offer a way of integrating psycho-oncological data. In fact, if we limit ourselves to the biomedical model we can hardly achieve an integrated understanding of cancer, which has a multidimensional aetiology (Baltrusch and Waltz 1985).

Stressful life events require increased efforts of adaptation on the part of the individual, and generally lead to painful states of tension; depending on the gravity of the situation, this may bring about the exhaustion of the capacity to fight, and to 'giving up'. For a physical illness to ensue, a synergy seems to be necessary between stress, the patient's personality structure and an unfavourable sociofamilial situation. Certain authors posit that external factors contribute to the direct induction of tumours and to the proliferation of cancerous cells, after exposure to a certain number of carcinogens (Sklar and Anisman 1980). Epidemiological studies have demonstrated, for example, that compared with the average for the population of the same age, widows or divorcées suffer more from depressive illness, cardio-vascular diseases and cancers (Weisman and Worden 1975, 1976–7). Some people have exhibited anomalies in the immune function after bereavement, with a significant diminution in the number of lymphocytes (Ader 1975; Dutz *et al.* 1976).

The richness of social relations plays a considerable part in the maintenance of the mental and physical health of the adult. It is clear that good-quality affective bonds are an essential factor in helping one to cope with difficult existential situations. Conversely, poor relationships, notably an undermined marital or family background, constitute a very unfavourable milieu. This is an argument which must be taken into account when caring for cancer patients, where a certain kind of pathology in relationships makes for difficulty. It is necessary to observe how the patient interacts with the therapeutic team, because that will be evidence of his early experiences of socialization. It is thus that the same factors that have hampered emotional development have played a not inconsiderable role in the pathogenesis of the disease and have influenced the cognitive and affective processes of response to stress and to cancer. All these aspects add up to the fact that in therapeutic practice one may well have to deal, without really being aware of it, with a natural selection of 'good' and 'bad' patients. In fact the most common tendency is to deal most and best with those who are at the least psychosocial risk. We have seen that the personal life-style of the patient, the manner in which he has led his life and been able to flourish, already give him effective adaptive resources and influence his prognosis. People who are inhibited, hyper-adapted, conformist, norm-fixated, and rejecting depression will create a corresponding attitude among the carers and render them inadequate or insufficient. It is for these people that a systematic programme of support must be developed.

THE PSYCHOBIOLOGICAL MODEL OF CANCER

The preceding pages show that we still have no fundamental understanding of the aetiology of neoplastic diseases at all levels of organization of the human being. The only certainty is that somatic mutation is an important factor, but is not a sufficient explanation for cancers (Greer and Watson 1985). More simply, one could say that there are mechanisms which control tumour growth and cellular dissemination, where the psyche certainly plays a protective role. Conversely, with certain individuals, psychological conflicts contribute to the emergence of cancers in synergy with biological disturbances. The role of stress has been mentioned (Greer and Morris 1975) but also contested (Schonfield 1975). One explanation of this contradiction is that often, in replying to questionnaires, patients are reluctant to admit that they have been through painful existential episodes. Moreover, retrospective studies introduce other uncertainties, because stories are reinterpreted. Enquiries often have recourse to psychometric tests which were originally established for psychiatric patients (the MMPI) and not tested on the very different population of cancer patients (Shekelle *et al.* 1981). Depressive antecedents, which often figure in the literature, may also be unreliable as a predictor (Greene 1966; LeShan 1966). Since the start of a cancer cannot be dated with accuracy, it is quite possible that depressive episodes were provoked by cancers already evolving but still undetected (Kerr *et al.* 1969) rather than by traumatic events. The only point of agreement is that there is some correlation between the diagnosis of cancer and a certain kind of behaviour characterized by abnormal control of aggression and affects (Bahnson and Bahnson 1966). The work of Greer demonstrates, for example, that women of under age 50 affected by cancer express less anger than members of a healthy control group of the same age (Greer and Morris 1975). According to another study, women who have had a mastectomy show their anxiety less, are apparently more optimistic and have a tendency to avoid conflicts (Jansen and Muenz 1984). Studies of melanoma have come to the same conclusions, with a discrepancy between the anxiety which is acknowledged, that is to say none, and that registered by electrodermal activity (Kneier and Temoshok 1984). But all is not yet clear. For certain people, emotional inhibition and the capacity to develop a cancer may both result from genetic factors and need not be in a causal relationship.

As with the personality of the coronary patient, there have been attempts to define a type 'C' behaviour typical of the cancer patient (Morris 1980). This is characterized principally, as seen above, by the inhibition of emotions and of aggressive reactions, as well as by conformism, exemplary submission, relationships without conflict, and patience. The importance of this profile is useful for indicating a prognosis. For melanoma, for example, this corresponds to the more invasive tumours (Temoshok 1985). A crucial element for behavioural research is that one would be dealing with suppression of behavioural responses rather than with repression of feelings (Greer and Watson 1985). In fact, in that study the subjects admitted having negative emotions but did not know how to find adequate behaviour to respond to them. Education certainly plays a very important role in 'C' behaviour, especially in the response to stress. For 'C' individuals, stressful situations are more threatening by reason of the control they exercise over themselves and their incapacity to utilize conflict as a model of reaction. Thus, despite an adequate perception of their emotion, they adopt a less effective and more rigid response (Pettingale *et al.* 1977).

According to classic behavioural models, it is acknowledged that perceived stress acts as a physiological trigger leading to the 'fight or flight' syndrome. The preparation of the body for the reaction may be demonstrated by measuring the increase in oxygen consumption and changes in muscle tone. Individuals who can speak about their feelings experience less stress at the physical level, for they quickly regain a state of equilibrium. A significant number of studies have shown that individuals who repress their emotions can only deal with stress by exercising increased physiological control. The question for cancer patients is to know whether type 'C' biological reactions have a pathogenic effect (Watson and Greer 1983).

Although suppression of emotion seems to play a part as much in psychosomatic ailments as in cancer, the precise mechanism of the action is not clear. In oncology, it could be true that the disease does not appear in response to the repetition of stressful events but depends on the specific biological and behavioural response that one brings to them. This hypothesis may be compared with the one which has been posited for individuals suffering from arterial hypertension. These patients present a specific problem of the autonomic pathways governing haemodynamics. All this would perhaps explain why it has not been possible to prove that cancer patients experience more stressful events than the general population. This is an encouragement to pursue research into the targets (the biological responses) rather than the effectors, whether stresses or events in their context.

The growth of the whole organism is under hormonal control. Psychological responses, particularly emotional reactions, produce alterations of tissues by limbic, hypothalamic, hypophysial, and endocrinological routes. Cancer is a disorder of the growth of cells which introduces a dysregulation of normal tissue balance. One could well imagine that psycho-endocrinological mechanisms play a part in the development of cancer. Up till now, there has been mostly talk of the immunological regulation of tumours, with the concept of immuno-surveillance and notably of the control of isolated cells of the NK (Natural Killer) type by psychological factors (Herberman 1982; Irwin *et al.* 1988; Bovbjerg 1989; Contrada *et al.* 1990).

If we admit the validity of type 'C' behaviour, we should research the biological variables associated with it. According to Greer (1984), for example, cancer patients showed exaggerated hormonal variation when faced with stress.

Chapter 2

Life turned upside down

'LAGTIME'

Many patients notice the first signs of illness several months or even years before they consult their doctor. Often they suspect that it may be cancer, particularly thanks to information they may have gathered from newspaper articles or television programmes. Some of them will react adequately by seeking medical advice. Others, up to 60 per cent of patients, will put off making an appointment (Henderson 1966). Often they have had experience of cancer among their family or friends, and life goes by as if the illness would not become a reality for them until formally diagnosed by a specialist. The most generally accepted explanation for this delay is that it allows them to build up defence and adaptation mechanisms (Gordon *et al.* 1980; Freidenbergs *et al.* 1981–2).

This is a period of getting used to the idea that their fate is about to change (Milton 1973). In other words, a certain delay can be a sign of adaptation to stressful situations. According to Weisman and Worden (1975), and taking a psychological viewpoint, this so-called lagtime is lengthened if defence mechanisms such as denial predominate and if there is social isolation, affective conflict and loss of hope for the future. On the other hand, there seems to be no connection with the type of tumour, except in the case of melanoma. Here the problem could be rather that the public has been ill-informed and has not known until recently how to recognize this type of tumour (Temoshok 1985). It seems that anxiety and depression, associated with denial, play a more important part in the refusal to consult a doctor than do more precise fears such as those of undergoing surgery or difficult treatment (Magarey *et al.* 1977). For others, the delay is a deliberate choice (Hackett *et al.* 1973).

The word 'delay' has taken on a pejorative connotation. Sometimes the doctor has difficulty in controlling his astonishment and says, 'Why didn't you come and see me sooner?'. The risk is that the patient will then feel criticized. This is why, if we take account of clinical, biological, and psychological factors, it is better to speak of 'free space' between the patient's discovery of his symptoms and his request for medical advice (Worden and Weisman 1980).

In fact, whatever we may say, the patient is not always wholly responsible for what happens. There is also the doctor's delay, the time that will elapse between the patient's first visit and the start of treatment. Sometimes the doctor himself does not assess the problem correctly. It is true that the symptom should first be carefully observed and subjected to a diagnostic process, which does not necessarily always point to the presence of a cancer. The symptoms of cancer of the stomach, for example, can be confused with peptic ulcers. But there are also all the doctor's fears, especially if he has a long relationship with his patient, which compound the subjective feelings of them both and lead to what we may call their 'shared denial'. This is their ability to agree that all is well, in the face of a situation which is too stressful to be confronted. This type of mechanism is known in other situations, for instance where there is a grave risk of suicide and the two protagonists are both agreed that all is well and there is no need for medical intervention or urgent hospitalization.

Many studies have tried to establish the psychosocial profile of the 'delayers'. But no significant correlation with cultural, intellectual, or socio-economic background has been established (Halman and Suttinger 1978).

At the time of the diagnosis, in order to explain the time which they have taken in coming to see the doctor, patients deny their fears and have recourse rather to rational explanations, such as: 'It couldn't happen to me'; 'It couldn't be cancer because there has never been any in the family'; or 'I haven't done anything to deserve it'.

Whatever the reasons for this delay may be, in the end everyone consults a doctor. The reason for this is that the patient has suddenly felt a change or a worsening of what he had already noticed, or his family has encouraged him, or the illness or death of a friend has made him take notice of the seriousness of the situation. Often, during the consultation, he asks questions about something irrelevant, some trivial symptom, or something that he has read. It is only towards the end of his appointment that he shows, by some turn of phrase, what is really worrying him. In these cases the doctor must totally avoid any expression of disapproval or disquiet. That could only strengthen the patient's feeling of guilt. This is also true for members of the family, who may feel responsible in not having observed matters more carefully or in not having insisted on the patient seeing the doctor.

To admit that one has delayed is also a way of establishing a relationship of trust, of consigning oneself to the doctor's competence. For the doctor, the most appropriate response is to accept the facts calmly, finding empathic words and making clear that cancer is a common disease. This exchange of truths leads to a reduction of the patient's fears, doubts, and mistrust, and serves to establish a good-quality doctor–patient relationship which will continue throughout the treatment.

FUNDAMENTAL FEARS

Once the diagnosis of cancer is made, the patient's whole life is upset, on affective, family, and sexual levels as well as regarding work and the socio-economic front. This will depend, of course, both on the patient's personality and on his past. Areas of conflict appear, associated both with the cancer and with the treatment which it requires. Whether it is a fact or his imagination, the patient will very soon feel that he belongs to a world apart, that he is misunderstood, even shunned. In contracting a disease with such a bad reputation, everyone will feel in his own way some fundamental fears (Morris *et al.* 1977; Maguire *et al.* 1978; Guex 1983), notably:

- *Fear of alienation.* The patient dreads, not so much death, which he finds hard to conceive, but abandonment, rejection, and isolation, especially at the beginning and the end of his illness. The severity of the treatment will reinforce his impression of being invaded and attacked, struck by an unjust fate, facing, all alone, the malaise of those around him and of the world of medicine (Bloom 1982; Carey 1974).
- *Fear of mutilation.* The cancerous invasion is felt as a significant attack on the integrity of the body, and threatens his self-image. The patient cannot easily envisage the treatment ahead (surgery, radiotherapy, or chemotherapy), which may involve changes in his

physical make-up or psychological functions, and also great suffering (Wortman 1984).

- *The sudden confrontation with his own vulnerability.* Even if the prognosis is favourable and gives hope of a good recovery, the limits of his life are now written down somewhere (Bronner-Huszar 1971). This violent upset on several levels sometimes gives rise to the need for assessment and allows feelings of guilt, thoughts of sins to be atoned for, or the desire to settle accounts which were previously pending. The most common symptoms are anguish, depression, hopelessness or helplessness (Schmale 1984), but they will depend greatly on his own resources or on those around him.

- *The fear of loss of control.* For many people, psychic equilibrium is ensured by the feelings of autonomy, usefulness, and influence which they acquired in adulthood. The appearance of an illness whose image and reputation are often more dramatic than its actual clinical manifestations brings a feeling of loss of control over one's own life. This feeling extends to the person himself, for there are many people who find it difficult to tolerate the change in their self-image, their worth, and their capability. The whole illness creates a problem of control. In fact, the origin of most cancers is still uncertain, since the disease can strike without advance warning and its development cannot be foreseen or controlled. It is very agonizing, even shattering for the patient, who, especially in the case of leukaemia, does not even have a specific area on which to focus his attention and energy (Miller *et al.* 1976; McIntosh 1974). The emotional reactions of those around him, which are often contradictory, the wealth of information at his disposal, and the need to escape from total dependence on the competence of others all reinforce this state (Klagsbrun 1970). Complete regression, or on the other hand hyperactivity or the choice of unorthodox treatments, may represent an attempt to regain control.

Such fears will be exacerbated from the time of the first consultations with the doctor. At the moment of diagnosis, and during the treatment, the patient will not only have to come to terms with the illness and the world of health care, often a new sphere, but will also have to fight to maintain a reasonable emotional balance and a satisfactory self-image, while retaining as far as possible good social and vocational integration. This task requires the mobilization of all the individual's ability to adapt, sometimes with the help of certain defence mechanisms which the doctor will have to acknowledge and respect, as long as they have a function. The presence of these mechanisms will often tend to give the impression that the patients do not feel properly understood or looked after (Legmen *et al.* 1978). They will be dissatisfied with the treatments and with the way that their families or carers communicate with them (Gordon *et al.* 1980). To a certain extent, this perception is borne out from the professional point of view; for example, the patient is often distanced (Feldman 1978). Out of 100 patients presenting with breast cancer who were asked about the reactions of their relatives to their condition, 72 felt a change of relationship and 50 felt avoided or feared (Peters-Golden 1982).

In street interviews, 66 per cent of people say that one must be above all optimistic and positive with cancer patients. Two-thirds of the patients themselves reply that they do not know how to handle this false optimism and that it gives them the feeling of being even more isolated (Cobb and Erbe 1978).

It is true that at the start of the illness the patient is very traumatized, but he still benefits from the energy, interest and hope of those around him. This changes with time and with the exhaustion of psychological and physical reserves. The time of diagnosis is one of great vulnerability for cancer patients: 20 to 50 per cent of people, according to the literature, show signs of depression, symptoms which are rarely expressed clearly but are recognizable by body language, somatic disorders, pains, unexpected side-effects of treatments, and a certain social or emotional withdrawal. The difficulty is that these symptoms are confused with the main clinical picture. Twenty-five per cent of these patients have cognitive disorders which are due not to cerebral metastases or psychological problems but to the so-called minimal side-effects of the treatments (Endicott 1984; Bahnson 1980).

ADAPTATION TO THE DISEASE

Adaptation to the disease consists of two main tasks:

– facing up to the disease itself, to all the problems which it gives rise to (psychosocial disruptions, pains, debility, etc.), coping with the treatments (restrictions, disagreeable side-effects), and developing satisfactory relationships with the medical team; and

– coming to terms with the alterations to one's life which have been brought about by the disease.

It is a question of keeping the best possible balance, of preserving clear relationships with the family circle and of preparing oneself to face an uncertain future (Singer 1984). Cobliner (1977), interviewing 300 women affected by gynaecological and breast cancers, established that successful adaptation to the disease was only possible on the basis of a set of positive personal and interpersonal factors, a good self-image and feeling of identity, confidence in medicine and in the effectiveness of the treatments, a spirit of openmindedness and readiness to engage with others, involvement in satisfying social activity, and a good correlation between one's expectations from life, the extent to which goals have been achieved, and the experience of overcoming previous existential crises.

Seeing through such a task to a successful conclusion varies according to the nature of the disease, the personality of patients, and the psychosocial conditions which surround them. One has the impression that adaptive capabilities are in inverse proportion to vulnerability. The most stable patients face up to reality, concentrate on positive aspects, and undergo treatments with confidence. The others, who have a poorer prognosis, have recourse to avoidance mechanisms, to passivity, to stoic submission. Suicide is rare, but it is also a possible strategy (Weisman 1976).

Certain studies have sought to establish if there is a preferred way of responding to stressful events (Ferlic *et al.* 1979; Morris *et al.* 1985). There are individual defence mechanisms, but it seems that people's behaviour is also conditioned by the circumstances in which they find themselves, whatever their perception of their own stress (Morris *et al.* 1985).

To keep his balance, the sick person therefore has at his disposal a certain number of resources that are bound up both with his individuality and with the situation: these are the Ego defence mechanisms and the mobilization of the family circle.

Reference has already been made above to the 'cancer personality'. It is important to avoid confusion in distinguishing adaptation to the illness from personality structure.

From a psychoanalytic and psychosomatic point of view, defence mechanisms are adjustments of personality that have perhaps played a part in the development of the disease and which a psychotherapeutic approach aims to modify. To speak of adaptation means, on the other hand, to assess how the individual, faced with a serious physical and psychic assault, uses his defence mechanisms as an effective protection, spontaneous and economical, in a situation where there is sometimes little else that can be done. Hackett and Cassem (1974) showed the importance of denial for the prolongation of survival in myocardial infarction and breast cancer. People who are 'healthy' make use of three types of strategy in confronting unpleasant events in everyday life:

- they try to change the situation (and so modify the stress);
- they try to change the meaning of the situation; and
- they try to control the stress by controlling themselves (Folkman *et al.* 1979; Pearlin and Schooler 1978).

It is around these three main points that defence against cancer and adaptation to it will be centred.

DEFENCE MECHANISMS: AN UNCONSCIOUS ADAPTATION TO ILLNESS

Denial consists of excluding from one's mind an intolerable problem or situation. The word implies the refusal to acknowledge reality, or its minimization. In fact, the cancer patient rarely denies the reality of his disease, as psychotics would do, but he prefers not to speak of it or not to confront it straight away, so as to give himself time to adapt to it.

Avoidance or *suppression* imply accepting reality while deliberately trying not to think about it.

These mechanisms are not, of course, static and quantifiable qualities. They are, rather, unconscious phenomena, more or less powerful according to the emotions experienced. These defences perhaps seem to be an escape, or self-delusion, but most often they offer time to mobilize intrapsychic resources and to build up other strategies for coping with the disease.

Projection soothes anguish and guilt, aggression or bad feelings by attributing to someone else or to an external cause the source of what is amiss. This is also a way of keeping the self-image intact by displacing the responsibility on to another target (the spouse or the doctor, for example). Aggression and the feeling of not enjoying the best possible care are connected.

Differential denial, or *selective ignorance*, show that often these mechanisms are not in watertight compartments constructed by the individual himself and for his sole use, but are rather an interactive process bound up with the situation. There are people who understand very well what is happening to them, but who think it necessary – in order to maintain a good relationship with their doctor (so as not to worry him or make too many demands on him), or to avoid torturing their families – to deny a part of their disease or their distress. Selective ignorance is the act of deliberately making a choice of positive elements at the heart of painful circumstances, allowing one to keep hope alive.

The problem is that this kind of functioning is very effective in reducing stress in everyday life, at work, and in contact with those to whom one has no emotional ties, whereas in family life it can increase tensions. In fact, relatives, if they are not given information, start to imagine things and have recourse to unsuitable solutions which show a certain lack of understanding. This also happens with doctors, who start to talk about what concerns them, death for example, when the patient has in his mind a much more immediate problem which he dares not mention.

Rationalizations are useful in defining a goal and giving meaning to the illness. These are often a reply to the piercing question 'why me?'. Perhaps this serves to allay guilt, one of the conceivable causes of cancer. For a wide public, the most functional explanation is that it is a question of a social ill and that its origin must be attributed to more general causes, such as living conditions, nutrition, or radioactivity, or more simply that it arises from the laws of chance. Attributing the onset of cancer to living conditions offers a rationale for choosing diets or adopting a more healthy way of life. It offers a framework for a radical change in life-style, which naturally depends on individual convictions. Finding a nutritional cause and following strict diets becomes an esoteric approach of transformation, by adopting a rigorous code of conduct which offers containment for anguish and uncertainty.

It is clear that defence mechanisms are not so much a denial of the disease as an opportunity for developing strategies for adaptation and values that reinforce hope or self-affirmation. They are also a path to follow in the face of many uncertainties.

Another way of coping is to engage in a more practical way with the external world, or to expect from it a more precise form of help. What we earlier called 'rationalizations' take the form of a demand for active collaboration with therapy, while wishing to know everything about the disease and its treatments. This intellectual mastery leads towards controlling the situation and sharing responsibility for the management of the illness.

After mutilating surgical interventions, there is also the opportunity to learn special re-education techniques: to join a group of volunteers for certain cancers or certain operations, such as groups for facial cancers, colostomy groups, or mastectomy groups. To prepare oneself to help others is not only to strengthen one's expertise and autonomy in relation to the doctors, but is also a way of sharing the knowledge and experience one has gained. The search for reassurance and emotional support among relatives, friends, the medical team and groups of volunteers allows the release of distress and tension. To aim for realistic goals, well defined, such as a return to part-time work or a holiday, is something simple and easy to achieve. The implicit goal is to escape from the unacceptable side of the global problem by breaking it down into limited tasks.

Adaptation to cancer necessitates using various resources and possibilities, following an order corresponding to the different stages in the development of the disease. To be thoroughly informed, by taking advice from several doctors, may give significant support at the time of diagnosis. At another stage, this might seem both inadequate and dangerous for the policy of care and a handicap to concentrating all forces on a specific task.

The central problem of this whole story is that of living constantly in uncertainty: to live with all the ambiguity of cancer, experienced as life-threatening but treated as a chronic sickness. Each person asks himself about the consequences, the risks of recurrence, the progressiveness of the disease and the anguish it will cause among family and friends. This uncertainty (this permanent feeling of insecurity) is the source of very exhausting contradictory feelings.

To sum up, in a somewhat simplistic manner, one might define adaptation to the disease as a complex process of searching for meaning, of challenge, and of working things out. Subjected to stress, and according to his own style of relating to the world, the patient will try to master the information, will modify his behaviour in line with his personality and his experience, and finally will adopt a strategy of adaptation. This is what has been called 'defensive evaluation'. In other words, a situation that is initially regarded as a threat sees its threatening nature buried in order to lessen the anguish that it provokes. The assessment of the external situation is thus constantly readapted by the stressed individual, according to the quantity of painful emotions that he can tolerate at any one time. It is a way of containing suffering within bearable limits. If the existential issues are too difficult to face, the patient will develop strategies centred on the immediate problem, seeking alone, or with the help of others, the practical resources which are directly applicable to the tasks in hand (Lazarus and Launier 1978; Folkman *et al.* 1979).

POOR ADAPTATION

We have seen that it was difficult to determine, with regard to cancer, a standard adaptative behaviour of the patient. The different studies which have attempted to do this had too restricted a brief and obtained only partial results (Holland 1977).

The gamut of human behaviour makes it equally difficult to know when there is a poor adaptation to the illness, with maladjusted defence mechanisms – in other words, to assess when an attitude becomes a real obstacle to effective therapy, compromising the prognosis. It is good, for example, that a patient denies a little the gravity of his state so that he accepts that he must fight, but not to the extent of losing his sense of reality. The signs of mal-adaptation should be spotted, and corrections to the course may be made if the relationship of trust between the patient and his relatives is good enough.

Farberow *et al.* (1964) have defined the main features of 'mal-adaptive syndrome'. This is revealed when the patient does not present the classical signs of rebellion on the announcement of his diagnosis (suffering, fear, and anger) (Wirsching *et al.* 1981).

Renneker (1981) has defined the 'pathological niceness syndrome'. This may signal dangerous ground and constitutes a risk factor. It is particularly important to monitor patients who present as too sub-missive, passive, and anxious in order to please the doctor (Bahnson 1976; Baltrusch 1975). Generally, they belong to the category of people who do not present any problem, and whom one appreciates for it, because they do not require one to devote too much time to them and are always in agreement.

Other signs are suggestive:

- an emotional reaction (depression, anxiety, defeatism, or a cog-nitive disorder) prevents the patient from asking for treatment or co-operating with it, or interferes with the treatment (Schonfield 1972; Morris *et al.* 1977);
- the patient's anxiety is the source of more suffering, pain, or side-

effects than the disease itself could give rise to (Meyerowitz 1979);
- emotional reactions hamper daily life (work, social interaction), or the individual gives up normal sources of gratification (for example, a patient becomes excessively dependent, while blocking therapeutic proposals, and shows a total dissatisfaction with the care he receives and the life he leads);
- psychiatric disorders appear, notably a collapse of self-esteem, and communication problems, with erroneous interpretations of all information; or threats of suicide, happily relatively rare, which always indicate a cry for help.

Of course, no general rule can be systematically applied and, as with all medical practice, each case must be individually assessed. Members of the health-care team should intervene to clarify the main difficulties or help the patients to find solutions by themselves if possible. One basic rule is to encourage them to speak about what they are going through, which is the only way of understanding them but also a way of making them *feel* understood.

It is clear that the seriousness of the disease, the site of the tumour, or the distinctive characteristics of the person will introduce factors of wide variability (Weisman and Worden 1976–7). We know that young patients are at risk, since they are at the age when questions of self-determination arise and emotional and vocational choices need to be made. For them, to be ill means to stop this evolution. People of more mature age, who have already accomplished one or more stages of their life with satisfaction, are more stable. The conjunction 'youth – high socio-economic level – physical disorders and poor prognosis' is prone to maladaptation (Craig and Abeloff 1974). Morris *et al.* (1977) found great emotional lability after breast amputation among women who had suffered depression in their childhood, and this independently of the circumstances of the diagnosis and treatment. A case history of anxiety and depression, before the illness or the operation, is an indication of future psychological difficulties (Jamison *et al.* 1978). On the other hand, presenting emotional problems at the time of the first manifestation of the disease is not a bad sign in itself. This shows that the patient can accept suffering and undergo a certain 'mourning for health' in an appropriate way and at the right time. Different studies (Maguire *et al.* 1978; Morris *et al.* 1977; Wellisch *et al.* 1985) have assessed the progress of a group of women five years after breast surgery.

They note that symptoms of anxiety/depression regress with time, from 46 per cent during the first weeks to 25 per cent at the end of one year and to 13 per cent after two years. Schonfield (1972), for his part, noted that nine months after their radiotherapy, 79 per cent of the patients examined had resumed work, and that there was a significant correlation with the level of anxiety and depression which had been noted at the time of the first assessment. This would mean that those who react emotionally in the most appropriate way at the outset become best reintegrated in everyday life.

We can sum things up as follows: adaptation is a constellation of many factors. It is necessary to observe and describe all that a person does during the difficult period to adapt to the changes in the situation. In this way one will be able to know if intervention is necessary or not and if surprises are in store for the future.

Self-assessment by the patient is rarely objective. It is therefore sometimes necessary to make enquiries from other sources, the nursing team, the doctor in charge, and the family, always seeking the patient's permission first.

As adaptive mechanisms are not static, one should not rely solely on a meticulous assessment but go with the flow and know that the patient may be different, may even be in contradiction with himself, according to the changes in his condition.

THE STAGES OF ADAPTATION TO THE DISEASE

Different attempts have been made to standardize the stages which the patient goes through in adapting to the disease and possibly preparing for a fatal outcome (Falek and Britton 1974; Kübler-Ross 1969). This analysis should be viewed with caution, for adaptation is specific to the patient and depends on a host of personal and contextual factors. Here too, the approach should be biopsychosocial, and one must acknowledge multiple adaptative tasks, fluctuating according to circumstances, but above all modulated by the relationships which the patient maintains with his relatives or with the medical team (Lipowski 1970). Greer et al. (1979) defined four ways of responding to stressful events: denial, fighting spirit, stoic acceptance, and helplessness/hopelessness, and to these was later added 'anxious preoccupation' (Moorey and Greer 1989; Greer et al. 1992).

This field has been particularly distinguished by the works of Kübler-Ross (1969, 1970), who has spoken of the stages in preparation for death. According to her, patients go through five distinct stages from diagnosis of terminal illness to their death. These comprise denial, anger, bargaining, depression, and final acceptance. The stage of acceptance is characterized by an absence of negative emotions such as depression and anger and a renunciation of the will to live. The patient no longer struggles against death and lives his last days peacefully. This concept, the fruit of Dr Kübler-Ross's wide personal experience, has great educational validity, for it compels care-givers to be aware of the non-linear and conflicting dynamic which a patient has to experience in order to end by accepting something extraordinary and unacceptable – death. However, one must not make a universal model out of this, and Kübler-Ross herself was surprised to see that a rigid scheme, with almost obligatory stages, had been drawn from it, even if they follow in a variable order. It is all the more striking if one sees that this has been transposed just as it is to the whole development of the disease, and not solely to the last stages. Some authors have called this observation into question (Pattison 1978; Schulz and Aderman 1974).

I should like to suggest rather that patients adopt a whole range of emotional response and appraisal of reality during the various stages of the disease. Some will make use of denial during the entire course of the illness. Others, after a period of denial, will become anxious and depressed. Perhaps the different stages are the result of a subtle process of socialization engendered by the family and the medical team. For example, a person can give the impression of denying, because he attunes himself to the mode of behaviour of those around him (this is what I called 'differential denial' above); that is to say, he denies reality only with certain people, often the doctor, but not with those with whom he feels trusted or understood.

Some patients never come to terms with the idea of having cancer, even if they live in long-term remission. This has been demonstrated by Silver and Wortman (1980), who noted that some people still remain anxious five to seven years after their diagnosis (Morris et al. 1977; Maguire et al. 1983) and after the end of their treatment, even with a high probability of cure. Reactions will also be very different according to people's age (Craig and Abeloff 1974; Plumb and Holland 1977).

The Kübler-Ross model poses a problem for the psychosocial approach to the cancer patient. For according to her the therapist should encourage the evolution of the patient through the different stages until acceptance of death has been achieved. One cannot adhere exclusively to this way of seeing things, for it is perhaps the doctor's idea that things should follow this progression. This may make him less receptive to the desires and wishes of the patient, who might well perhaps want to do otherwise. Worse, one might even come to consider the patient who refuses a peaceful death as pathological. It is not necessarily more desirable to be silent at the moment of death, instead of crying out one's anguish, depression, or denial. It is quite clear that given the present possibilities of palliative care for patients in hospital, medical teams prefer peaceful people who do not create an upheaval of ward routines but instead suffer in silence.

There are several ways of living, as there are several ways of dying, and practitioners should be concerned less with knowing how patients *ought* to die than with how they *want* to die (Lazarus and Launier 1978).

THE LIFE CYCLE AND CANCER

Attitude and adaptation to the disease will be very different according to the age of the patient.

For the young adult, life is full of potential. It is the time of beginnings, starting work or a training course, marriage and children. It is the time of financial obligations and increased responsibilities. Illness is going to upset this period of choice and postpone the taking of a certain number of decisions, which perhaps may never offer themselves again. Moreover, young people are not used to being ill; quite the contrary, their energy and their good physique have given them a certain feeling of invulnerability; they are not at all inclined to take care of themselves or pamper themselves.

Being ill entails a feeling of loss and the necessity of accepting that one must renounce certain dreams and plans. If the young adult is still in the phase of growing up, cancer is going to represent a considerable setback for him, and perhaps entail the calling into question of acquired roles and the interruption of new and still fragile relationships. Parents will perhaps regain their power over him and he will find himself once again in the position of dependence which he has just left behind. If he or she is recently married, the partner will suddenly have to take on tasks that are too heavy, which (s)he is perhaps not prepared for and lacks the maturity to tackle. Unmarried people will ask themselves many emotional questions, worrying about not being able to have normal love affairs because of physical handicaps, and aesthetic and sexual problems.

Even for a healthy individual, middle age is a period of physical and relational changes which demands great psychological flexibility. This is the stage of the 'empty nest', which comes along when the children are grown up and the grandparents die. Successful adaptation involves renewing the bonds between the couple and engaging in extrafamilial activities. If someone, because of his illness, is handicapped in tackling this stage properly, he risks going through it much more dramatically, for example by trying to cling onto his children or prevent them from growing up. This is also the case for those who have invested everything in their professional career or in their social success and who suddenly find themselves isolated, without other resources or abilities to tackle stressful events with a modicum of emotional stability.

Old people have to accept their age and get used to the idea of death. The time has come for them to try to give meaning to what they have experienced and to draw up a balance sheet. This implies that a certain degree of serenity and satisfaction has been reached, and that one can accept that agonizing feeling that time is now too short to correct past mistakes or begin a new life. Without fail, cancer will remind one of one's limits, and if existential goals have not been achieved, it may be the cause of a serious depressive syndrome, indeed a complete decline.

To be old also means a modification of one's image of oneself and one's body, which it is not always easy to accept. For patients who refuse to see themselves growing old or who have not yet realized that they have entered into this stage of life, the diagnosis of cancer has every chance of brutally pushing them into it. To the trauma of the illness will be added, then, the sudden realization that time has run out. Other patients, on the other hand, who have accepted that they have come to the end of their time, will not take the discovery at all badly, since they will easily understand that it will not greatly affect their chances of survival.

Chapter 3

The concept of 'quality of life'

GENERAL

The impact that the disease and the treatments have on the quality of life is of interest as much to care-givers as to patients and their relatives (de Haes and van Knippenberg 1985; Wellisch 1984). Advances in treatment have had the result – cancer often now being a chronic disease – that it is more a question of knowing how to survive rather than how to prepare for a fatal outcome. The policy of care must go beyond the traditional biomedical procedures and be concerned with total well-being (Fallowfield 1990). The treatments are aggressive in their impact on the physical, social, and emotional life of patients (Greer 1984). Surgery is at times very mutilating (breast, ENT area, urogenital system and rectum); radiotherapy has significant secondary effects (skin problems, postactinic lesions, asthenia, anxiety and depression) (Priestman *et al.* 1981); chemotherapy, often considered to be the most disturbing, is administered over long periods and induces considerable toxicity (nausea, vomiting, digestive problems, hair loss, and anxiety) (Linssen *et al.* 1982; Priestman and Baum 1976; Hochberg and Linggood 1979). It is necessary to assess whether the chances of improvement and survival have any benefit in comparison with all the inconveniences. For most writers, the concept of quality of life is more important than quantity and duration. It integrates physical comfort, psychological well-being, and level of performance. It should be linked with an assessment of the wider social context and function. Moreover, the economic aspect should not be neglected, since some patients often devote large sums to the search for adjuvant treatments and special diets to alleviate their distress.

The quality of life should be the subject of research set out under several headings:

- the reactions of the patient to the cancer and the treatments;
- the correlation between the different reactions and the average quality of life;
- the comparison of the respective costs and benefits of the treatments (for example, if two treatments offer the same survival rate, one must choose the one that offers the greater comfort);
- the recording of the patient's complaints, which should influence the attitudes of therapists and lead to a better understanding of his overall needs.

Various studies have described the effect of chemotherapy on life and behaviour (Meyerowitz 1980). Vera (1981) noted that we had totally neglected the sexual problems of patients who had undergone gynaecological surgery and who appeared well adapted to life. Radiotherapy is a source of anxiety, but it affects the sexuality of prostatic patients less than surgery (Leibel *et al.* 1980). Thus one gets a false picture of the quality of life. Contrary to what one might think, the amputation of a leg attacked by a sarcoma, followed by chemotherapy, is not less popular than a conservative approach associated with radiotherapy (Sugerbaker *et al.* 1982).

Enquiries made among patients sometimes do not give the expected results. Where one would expect a negative effect of the treatment one finds little difference in quality of life between groups of patients and groups of healthy people, if one takes no account of the view that each one has of his quality of life (Nou and Aberg 1980). According to Helson and Bevan (1967), a person's level of adaptation corresponds to the locus of experiences of life, past and present. It will continually change according to new data. Thus the well-being of patients may be modulated by the experience they already have of the disease, by the type of doctor–patient relationship, but also by their attitude in the face of cancer. The quality of life is then the resultant of the different elements entering into the balance-sheet. For some patients, the disadvantages of the disease are compensated for by certain new and positive aspects which they experience both in their bodies and in relation to their families (Meyerowitz 1980). For others, it is perhaps a traumatic experience, but one which at the same time brings into awareness unknown aspects of their inner resources.

NAUSEA AND VOMITING

Many patients have nausea and vomiting in the course of their illness. These symptoms are due to the direct effect of the illness (cerebral metastases, digestive obstructions, metabolic disorders) or that of the treatments. These are continuous or episodic manifestations (dehydration, malnutrition, debility, isolation), controllable or uncontrollable, which disturb social and physical activities.

Nausea and vomiting induced by chemotherapy are the most often quoted, because this is one of the main forms of treatment. One often observes behavioural changes that give rise to side-effects well before the administration of the treatments, leading to refusal of therapy, and much anxiety and depression (Stoudemire *et al.* 1984; Seigel and Longon 1981; Weddington 1982; Whitehead 1975).

These behavioural changes are linked with the fact that people know that the drugs used are toxic not only for the cancerous growths but also for normal tissues (Burish and Bradley 1983; Golden 1975). The presence or absence of nausea and vomiting depends on the chemical agents used and the efficacy of anti-emetics. Doxorubicin and cisplatin are very emetic, while fluorouracil and vincristine are less so. Like painkilling drugs, anti-emetics should be prescribed with knowledge of the effective doses and the response of patients. Trial and error are sometimes necessary. Often, patients' compliance is poor because one allows them to judge the dose to take according to the seriousness of their symptoms, and they are afraid of overdosing themselves.

The duration and the intensity of nausea and vomiting which appear after chemotherapy are variable (Morrow 1984; Fetting *et al.* 1982). Sometimes the symptoms anticipate the treatments. In fact, some patients feel sick when merely thinking about their chemotherapy the day before the treatment, on the way to the hospital, or encountering the smells or colours of the treatment room. This anticipatory nausea is the result, as with chronic pain, of a process of classical conditioning (Bernstein *et al.* 1979). Repeated injections of cytotoxic chemicals in association with contextual stimuli (smells, sounds, colours) give rise to the development of nausea and vomiting, which in their turn make the response worse. This is the experience of 25 to 50 per cent of patients. Their general characteristics are that they are young, have already undergone a number of courses of treatment (Fetting *et al.* 1983), are anxious (Ingle *et al.* 1984) and emotional (Nerenz *et al.* 1982), and have had violent vomiting and nausea at the time of their first treatment. This last factor appears to be the most significant indicator of the risk of later developing anticipatory side-effects. Patients must always be reassured, by making clear to them that they are not responsible for what happens, that it is an automatic and normal response which is quite involuntary.

In radiotherapy, too, nausea and vomiting are frequent, according to the dose of radiation and the area of the body treated, especially in the case of the abdomen (Welch 1980).

Behavioural therapy methods are the techniques of choice for dealing with these problems, centred on the symptom, aiming to break the effective circuit of the anticipatory side-effects – that is to say, those that take place even before the administration of the treatments (Redd *et al.* 1982a; Redd 1982b; Redd and Andrykowski 1982c).

ALIMENTARY DISORDERS

The impairment of the desire to eat (anorexia) and the accompanying loss of weight may occur at each stage of the illness, to varying degrees. They have various causes: a transient anorexia due to psychological shock at the time of the diagnosis, a secondary anorexia at the time of treatment, and loss of appetite due to the progression of the disease. In the early stages of cancer, psychic disorders show themselves particularly by a lessening of appetite. The diagnosis is an assault on the patient, making him fear for the integrity of his body and for his life. Chemotherapy may also bring with it alimentary disorders, particularly chemicals such as cyclophosphamide, nitrogen mustards, procarbazine, dactinomycin and cisplatin. Loss of appetite is often the first emotional response to an anxiety-provoking atmosphere. Patients may remember that their illness began with a lessening of appetite and weight loss; every fear of recurrence may well show itself for them in the same way. Anorexia is often associated with a state of depression. Certain studies show that depression among cancer patients is manifested by feelings of low self-worth, uselessness, and guilt. Functional disorders, generally associated with latent depression, are difficult to distinguish in cancer patients from progression of the disease: anorexia, weight loss, insomnia, excessive tiredness, diminution of libido, and loss of interest in daily tasks (Holland and Mastrovito 1980). Cachexia (general debility) is the most usual nutritional complication, characterized by loss of weight and dissolving of tissue. The mechanism of this is poorly understood; it may be a direct effect of the tumour (for example, in the case of cerebral or abdominal metastases) or of its treatments (DeWys 1979). The most obvious cause is a lessening of the supply of calories and proteins due to the treatments, pain, and nausea and vomiting, but it may also be a consequence of the alteration of taste (with ENT tumour or radiotherapy). It may also arise from an alteration of intestinal function, of the metabolism of proteins, fats and carbohydrates, or from an inhibition of the centres of hypothalamic control by tumoral metabolites (Theologides 1972). Since appetite and nutritional needs are also partly of reflex origin, behavioural cycles are triggered when certain foods or tastes are directly associated with aspects of the disease (Redd *et al.* 1982a; Redd 1982b; Redd and Andrykowski 1982c). One should avoid talking about digestive problems but rather encourage the absorption of small quantities of food, chosen from the patient's favourite dishes. A good way of working is to associate the taking of food with relaxation and to present it in an attractive and tempting way.

At St Christopher's Hospice in London, good results have been obtained by allowing the members of the family to share the patient's meals, or in trying to reintroduce the patient's usual foods (Saunders 1982).

Apart from specific alimentary disorders, the general deterioration in health may make the regular intake of food difficult. Fatigue will prevent the patient from going shopping, preparing meals, or eating them. If one skimps the careful preparation of dishes, meals will inevitably be less attractive.

SEXUAL PROBLEMS

Patients do not usually ask about the impact of their disease on their sexual function. Doctors avoid the subject and prefer to interpret the absence of questions as a good sign of adaptation. In fact, many people admit, if one questions them, that their sexual activity has diminished or even stopped after their cancer (Rosenthal and Kaufman 1974). The main reason is that because of physical problems, patients often feel undesirable and devalued. They experience their illness as a brake on their sexual expression or at any rate an obstacle to physical contact, which would offer them the warmth and comfort that they need. It is important to maintain sexual activity as far as possible, for libido summons up vital energy and is opposed to the picture of cancer as a debilitating condition, characterized by apathy, weakness, and giving up.

Even after hysterectomies for benign conditions, an increased number of sexual disorders are encountered (Derogatis and Kourlesis 1981a; Derogatis *et al.* 1981b, 1983); the problem is still more serious after more extensive pelvic surgery, where these problems are significant for women who have otherwise resumed a normal existence (Andersen and Hacker 1983; Holland and Mastrovito 1980). The seriousness of the illness plays a part, as well as the sexual experiences and the quality of affective relationships that existed formerly (Wise 1979). Of course, fatigue, physical disorders, pain, or anxiety limit the physical possibilities of patients, even if their desire is intact. There is no general epidemiological study on the sexuality of cancer patients. Most of the studies have analysed particular groups of patients whose disease has affected a sexual organ: the breast (Bransfield 1982–3; Silberfarb *et al.* 1980a; Jamison *et al.* 1978), the gynaecological area (Capone *et al.* 1980; Vincent *et al.* 1975; Sewell and Edwards 1980; Chapman *et al.* 1981), and the testicles (Schilsky *et al.* 1980). But the problem is wider, and is not confined to genital cancers.

Sexual dysfunction linked with cancer has several causes. We must distinguish the physiological aspects from the psychological.

The lowering of the level of sexual hormones due to treatment (cyproterone acetate is an example) brings with it a lessening of libido, and desire decreases. Sometimes this is a help, because it does away with sexual frustrations. On the other hand, if someone receives hormone therapy, in particular testosterone, for a metastatic breast cancer, increased desire and an improved sexual function may arise just when physical difficulties make all sexual relations impossible (in the case of pain, for example, or asthenia).

A depressed patient may exaggerate his complaints, or his lack of sexual interest, when his libidinal potentiality is intact.

Sexual behaviour is multifactorial: somatic, psychological, and relational. A diminution of libido induced by chemotherapy may produce anxiety, low self-esteem and the fear of rejection. The partner will be afraid of upsetting his spouse by broaching the subject; he will feel guilty or will assume that he must forgo all sexual relations, when such behaviour is ill-adapted to the state of the disease and the actual prognosis (Derogatis *et al.* 1981a, 1981b).

Apart from the effect of the cancer on sexual function, the problem must be faced of the sterility of young patients treated, for example, for testicular cancers, Hodgkin's disease, or the leukaemias.

The doctor must ask himself various questions:

- If someone is starting chemotherapy, can one reply to his questions on his future sexual life and his fertility?
- If one has the choice of two treatments, will one take into consideration which will do the least damage to the sexual function?
- Are the disorders brought about by the treatments potentially reversible or avoidable (should one think, for example, of banking sperm for a young man?) (Chapman 1979; Thachil et al. 1981)?
- When sexual problems occur, are there ways of treating them?

We must always analyse the causes of dysfunction and treat the disorders, which are both emotional and organic. At any rate, the patient should be informed and should be encouraged to talk about his problems, for he will rarely broach them of his own accord.

Certain surgical techniques may sever the nerves that are essential to erection and ejaculation (Thachil et al. 1981). A cystectomy or a prostatectomy, a retroperitoneal lymph-node dissection for a seminoma, may have this effect. Certain types of chemotherapy, such as vincristine or bleomycin, may lead to an autonomic neuropathy with constipation, urinary problems, and impotence (Rosenthal and Kaufman 1974; Schilsky et al. 1980).

Cancer treatments generally affect fertility (often temporarily but up to three years after certain radiotherapy treatments) but more rarely libido. Young women are not affected on a long-term basis by relatively high doses of radiation to the pelvic area, but 600 centigrays are enough to induce a menopause among women over age 40 (producing ovarian fibrosis and follicular destruction) (Thomas et al. 1976). The oestrogen deficiencies that result bring about the usual disorders of the climacteric, such as hot flushes, vaginal dryness, and dyspareunia. Chapman et al. (1981) observed that 25 per cent of patients in this category were involved in divorces or separations.

At the psychological level, reactions can arise in various ways. Many studies have been made of women who have had mastectomies. They often have sexual problems, which are bound up with the change in their feminine identity and the assault on their body image (Bronner-Huszar 1971; Silberfarb 1984a; Schain 1982). Breast cancer patients often show symptoms associated with hormonal changes, whether as a result of hormone therapy (tamoxifen), chemotherapy (doxorubicin, cyclophosphamide, methotrexate, vincristine), radiotherapy, or, among premenopausal women, oophorectomy. These are hot flushes, paraesthesia (itching or burning, pins and needles), mood swings, fatigue, headaches, and insomnia. The alteration of sexual function is associated with a lack of vaginal lubrication or expansion and with a loss of orgasm. Certain remedies seem effective in dealing with these drawbacks, such as lubricant jelly, vaginal dilators, and also magnesium or adrenergics (Silberfarb et al. 1980a). In marital relationships, Jamison et al. (1978) have shown that 23 per cent of women experienced a serious impact on their sex life, that 30 per cent of spouses underestimated the effect of the operation, and that 18 per cent were sexually unsatisfied.

Capone et al. (1980) have assessed the effectiveness of individual counselling offered to patients recently treated for a gynaecological cancer. Psychological distress, sexual functioning, and the return to work were assessed three, six, and twelve months after the interviews. The group of patients offered help were compared to a similar group left to themselves. Capone noted that, three months after treatment, the supported patients showed less alteration of their body image. On the other hand, the two groups were similar with regard to maintaining sexual activity and employment. After a year, the women who had been able to speak about their sexual problems seemed to have regained a more satisfying functioning than the others.

Certain authors have noted that emotional reactions to the loss of a testicle were considerably weaker than one might expect among young patients; nevertheless, after the end of treatment, 30 per cent of them had significant psychosocial disorders, even leading to psychological illness (problems at work and in emotional and family relationships) (Guex et al. 1983).

The last factor contributing to sexual problems is linked with the reaction of the partner, who may refuse sexual relations because of repugnance or fear of hurting the patient. In an enquiry among the husbands of mastectomy patients, Jamison et al. (1978) showed that 20 per cent of them had never seen their wives naked after their surgery. In certain cases, this phenomenon was attributed to the distaste of the husband rather than the shame or the discomfort of the patient.

In conclusion, sexual dysfunction in connection with cancer may have emotional and psychological ramifications. For many individuals, a satisfying sex life represents a reinforcement of identity, gratification, and self-esteem. Consequently, sexual dysfunction may lead to a state of depression and an impoverishment of the quality of life. This alters the relationships with partners and increases the degree of isolation.

These difficulties may also dissuade the patient from continuing his treatment, if his quality of life falls below a tolerable threshold. Certain patients will ask for a less aggressive treatment or will discontinue it rather than deprive themselves of a sex life (Vincent *et al.* 1975).

DEPRESSION

Depressive symptoms are frequent among cancer patients (Endicott 1984). The prevalence varies from 23 per cent (Plumb and Holland 1981) to 56 per cent (Levine *et al.* 1978) according to the literature. Derogatis *et al.* (1983) discovered major depressive episodes in 6 per cent, problems of adaptation in 12 per cent, and anxio-depressive symptoms in 13 per cent of 250 out- and in-patients drawn from three different cancer treatment centres.

One of the great difficulties in diagnosing a state of depression in a cancer patient is that of distinguishing it from the secondary manifestations of the disease or its treatments (Endicott 1984).

Major depressive episodes

According to the DSM IIIR classification (the psychiatric nomenclature of the American Psychiatric Association), depression is characterized by, among other things, loss of appetite, asthenia, insomnia, and physical disorders. For the cancer patient, it is difficult to know if a depressive state is actually of emotional origin or if it is secondary to an organic pathology, or both. In any case, it is impossible to assess a cancer patient using the same criteria as for psychiatric patients. It is best not to make a differential diagnosis between organic and functional disorders, but to accept the syndrome, as soon as the patient presents a state compatible with the changes of mood and behaviour attributable to psychopathology.

We must remember that the psychological state (for example, anxiety, depression, or phobia) can be caused or aggravated by the medical situation. This does not of course exclude the making of traditional diagnoses for depressive states pre-existing the cancer.

To determine a state of depression there must have been a change of mood or a persistent loss of interest for at least a week, so as to avoid classifying everybody as depressive. It is often necessary to make the diagnosis oneself, for many patients do not easily accept the idea that they are depressive and follow literally the instructions they receive not to show any negative thought (we may term this 'psychosomatic adjustment').

The clinical signs are apparent in the facial expression, the drooping features, the look of being near to tears, the body language (drooping shoulders, slowed-up movements, lowered eyes), the social withdrawal, the pessimistic remarks or the negative feelings. Complementary factors are irritability, poor acceptance of treatments, refusal of visitors or of activities. It is helpful to have the opinion of the family, who will perhaps have noticed changes in interest, a hypersensitivity, suicidal thoughts, or an unaccustomed calm. A personal or family history of previous depressive episodes is an increased risk factor, as is a history of other mental disorders or alcoholism. The problem with the diagnosis of depression is that often one projects on to the patient one's own feelings of despair with regard to cancer. There are, moreover, certain advantages in making such a diagnosis. There are pharmacological interventions for depression, whereas one is perhaps less equipped to deal holistically with the patient's well-being. Depression is sometimes associated with increased pain or with new pains, which complicate the clinical picture. Depressives are resistant to treatment, for they think that no one can help them. Moreover, the aggressiveness associated with depression alters the family atmosphere and relationships with the health-care team, with the risk of isolating the patient. But one must avoid abusing this diagnosis, so as not to complicate the treatment unnecessarily or miss a recurrence by misinterpreting changes in appetite and fatigue (Goldberg and Tull 1983).

Maladjustment disorders

These are less obvious on the clinical front and possibly correspond with latent depression. They are more connected with socio-occupational, relational, or illness-related problems, and respond less to psychotropic drugs. One may put them in the category of the reactions of grief or of depressive anxiety, arising after the diagnosis of the illness, after a recurrence, or on the unforeseen resumption of treatment. Grieving is characterized by intermittent depressive elements.

'Toxic' symptoms

The state of depression may result from cerebral metastases, from a tumour in the temporal lobe, from thyroid malfunction, or from cancer of the pancreas, among other sites. Other sources are possible, such as a general toxic reaction to medication, hypercalcaemia (Segaloff 1981), hepatic impairment (Schafer and Jones 1982), an endocrine disorder (Segaloff 1981), psycho-active tumours (Brown and Paraskevas 1982), or some other metabolic problem (Goldberg and Tull 1983).

In general, depression in cancer patients, whatever form it takes, is treatable by antidepressant medications, if these do not interact too much with the basic cancer treatment, but these should not be prescribed automatically, before any attempt at counselling or psychotherapy.

PSYCHOTIC SYMPTOMS

One must watch out for difficulties in the perception of reality or for hallucinations associated with a depressive state. These psychotic symptoms are either bound up with the personality of the patient or they are exogenous, arising from the physical disease or the medical treatments. In the latter case, the hallucinations will be visual rather than auditory. The risk of suicide is significant just when the picture of depression begins to improve. This clinical conjunction poses problems of care; patients may be angry, over-suspicious, or afraid that they will be harmed or poisoned. They refuse food and treatment and have a strange and disorganized way of rebelling against therapy, of tearing out their drip or of leaving the treatment room without explanation.

If the patient has a case history of bipolar depression (alternating phases of mania and depression), one must not forget to maintain the basic treatment, if it is compatible with the care of the present illness. One must think of it if there is irritability, agitation, reduced need for sleep, expansiveness, or grandiose manifestations.

COGNITIVE DISORDERS

Alterations in mental state are observed fairly frequently during the course of the disease (Folstein *et al.* 1984). Doctors must assess the capacity of the patient to give an adequate case history, to understand the situation in which he finds himself, and to consider the information he is given about his illness and its treatment. Cognitive disorders are often observed among hospitalized patients at an advanced stage of the disease: one study (Silberfarb et al. 1980b) showed that a quarter of such patients suffered from a more or less serious cognitive disorder. They had problems with memory, concentration, reasoning and judgement, sometimes even confusion and disorientation in space and time. Behavioural disorders may here be associated with disturbances of diurnal rhythm, irritability, changes in character, or an alteration in psychomotor activity. The patient oscillates between excitation and stupor. To sum up, one may distinguish four sources of cognitive problems:

– mental retardation (shown by the patient's history);
– focal cerebral lesions, due to metastases or to a cerebral tumour, with a corresponding neurological picture;
– dementia (personality changes with apathy, social withdrawal, loss of memory and spatio-temporal disorientation);
– exogenous psychoses (Engel and Romano 1959; Bonhoeffer 1974; Tune *et al.* 1981).

Exogenous psychosis may be characterized by drowsiness and other disorders of the level of consciousness (Stiefel et al. 1989). The clinician then has the impression that the patient is out of reach and that he must be stimulated, verbally or by touch, to obtain a response. Other disorders may be present, such as a lessening of attention and of concentration, disorders of memory recall and fixation, an alteration of comprehension and of perception, a modification of psychomotor activity (increased or reduced), and, in certain extreme cases, hallucinations. For the most part, these disorders are due to metabolic disturbances or to the direct effect of the tumour, including:

– primary toxins produced by the tumour;
– hypercalcaemia, hepatic impairment, electrolyte imbalance, thrombotic endocarditis (Reagan and Okazaki 1974; Bartuska 1975; Weisman and Sobel 1979; Webb and Gehl 1981).

The toxic effect of certain medications has been noted, in particular chemotherapy (procarbazine, fluorouracil, vincristine, methotrexate, and doxorubicin). The effect of corticosteroids, which can give rise to hallucinations or manic states, is well known (Stiefel *et al.* 1989).

The impact of radiotherapy has been less well assessed. One study has demonstrated problems with school work, linked with memory disorders and lack of attention and concentration, among children and adolescents with acute lymphoblastic leukaemia who underwent prophylactic cerebral radiotherapy (Soni *et al.* 1975).

It must be mentioned that certain cognitive disorders have nothing toxic or exogenous about them but are linked to psychological problems. Many patients, in fact, present a vulnerable personality and a high degree of existential distress before the onset of the disease. The eruption of cancer and its procession of traumas may therefore act as a precipitating factor for the problems described above.

It must be remembered that hypnotic medications, the benzodiazepines and narcotic analgesics, may all give rise to cognitive changes which are, however, reversible after a modification of the dosage (Silberfarb 1984a).

ANXIETY

There are few diseases that provoke as much anxiety as cancer. Many studies have tried to estimate the prevalence of anxiety among cancer patients (Lee and Maguire 1975; Morris *et al.* 1977; Derogatis *et al.* 1983; Gottschalk 1984). Unfortunately, as for certain depressive states, anxiety is a subjective phenomenon that is very difficult to evaluate by a research methodology, though some attempts to do so have been made (Zigmond and Snaith 1983; de Haes *et al.* 1990). The fears most commonly associated with cancer include the fear of death and of the unknown, of suffering, losing control, and being abandoned. There are more specific worries, connected with the sites of the disease or the types of treatment undergone. We have already spoken of the psychological after-effects of mastectomy, which affect sexual identity and body image (Meyerowitz 1980). These characteristics are also found with ear-nose-and-throat, gynaecological, and genito-urinary cancers. During the entire course of his disease, the patient will have to face great uncertainties and much stress, which causes anxiety. This is the case, for example, during the periods of waiting for a diagnosis or for the result of biopsies or laboratory tests. Anxiety is at its height, also, when a therapeutic protocol is broken off and the patient finds himself once again without treatment and free of all symptoms. He will then easily feel abandoned and will present functional manifestations, which may be expected to guarantee continuing therapy (Gorzynski and Holland 1979; Krant 1981). The fear of recurrence is certainly an anxiogenic state, one with which the patient is most often confronted (Silberfarb *et al.* 1980b).

Therapeutic strategies and diagnostic techniques, such as lumbar or bone-marrow punctures, are also the source of many worries on the part of the patient (Katz *et al.* 1980). Chemotherapy and radiotherapy are anxiogenic in so far as patients learn quickly that they produce relatively rapid adverse effects. Freidenbergs *et al.* (1981–2) have noted that in radiotherapy the use of a quiet machine like the betatron allays anxiety and depression. Anxiety is at the root of the anticipatory nauseas encountered in chemotherapy (Redd *et al.* 1982a; Redd 1982b; Redd and Andrykowski 1982c). In these cases, the patients describe how they are overcome by fear and anxiety several days before the expected procedure. It is the same when it is a matter of finding a good vein, at the moment of inserting the drip, or when the nurse 'who is good at injections' is not there. Anxiety is one of the constituent factors of the behavioural conditioning described in the section 'Nausea and vomiting' above (Spence 1964).

Anxiety is at the root of patients' refusal of treatment, or of their desire to change the regime, to escape what they feel to be threatening. This may be an indication of loss of confidence in medicine, which may bring with it the interruption of treatment and the recourse to adjuvant therapies.

Chapter 4

The pain of the cancer patient

ACUTE AND CHRONIC PAIN

Pain is an important symptom in oncology. Many patients will suffer it at some time during the course of their illness. Of course it depends on the site or the type of tumour, but also on the therapeutic methods utilized and the psychosocial context in which the disease occurs (Foley 1982; Payne and Foley 1984). Certain tumours have few painful symptoms, such as lymphoma or leukaemia (only 10–20 per cent), while others are much more painful, notably those of the skeleton and the ENT area (80 per cent) (Bonica 1979). The prevalence of pain increases with the severity of the illness (Twycross and Fairfield 1982); 60 to 90 per cent of patients with advanced cancer complain of it (Cleeland 1984), and often at this stage the main palliative is to ensure pain control (Saunders 1982).

Pain is a complex phenomenon, associated with actual or potential tissue lesions, but it is also influenced by the emotions, the culture, and the existential circumstances of the patient. These elements play an important part, whether the pain is acute or chronic, but they should be borne in mind above all when it is chronic (Degenaar 1979). Acute pain is a warning mechanism that alerts one to the fact that something is amiss in the organism. The stimuli can be identified, the lesion treated, and a period of improvement anticipated. But if the symptom persists, without new somatic elements to complicate the issue, then one speaks of chronic pain (Sternbach 1974; Melzack et al. 1985). At this point we must think of another dimension to the problem: the pain may well have a different function (Eich et al. 1985), and it is important to understand this, for it will influence the patient's response to analgesia. If the pain has been effective, for example, in attracting attention within a relationship, the patient will give it up with difficulty, unless one offers him an alternative (Guex 1986b). Assessing chronic pain requires a comprehensive approach to the problem, or taking into account the multiple factors that go to make it up. It is known that the therapeutic methods usually employed to ameliorate acute pain are of no use for chronic pain, and that they may even make the symptom worse (Guck *et al.* 1985). In general, the patient in chronic pain and his relatives establish and maintain behaviours that are bound up with the disease. The suppression of the symptom does not allow a return to the former state. One must speak, then, of 'operant behaviours', for the interactions between the patient and his family or his doctor will often reinforce the symptom (Turner and Chapman 1982). A stimulus provokes a certain type of behaviour (for example stopping work, an analgesic medication, or additional care). If, for one reason or another, the persistence of the pain is necessary, and if it always results in the same type of consequence (for example, more assiduous care from the doctor), it will therefore also come to depend on the consequences, which then reinforce the symptom. For certain patients, it is difficult to know if they take analgesics because they have pain or if they have pain because analgesics soothe them. The only way of breaking this vicious circle is to analyse the factor giving rise to the reinforcing effect. In chronic cases, everything takes effect very quickly, even the type of communication employed with the patients. One must endeavour to avoid this type of interaction by trying to observe what the patient does rather than what he says or registers openly, for what he says will anticipate the response he expects. If someone says that he cannot get up because he has pain, one must understand that he cannot get up and not try to explain why he cannot get up, because the cause that could be treated is often no longer present. It is always possible to envisage what can be changed or ameliorated, in spite of the pain, or what means can be made available to gain a very small percentage of activity. It is clear that this is very different from acute pain, which temporarily involves clinical manifestations and analgesic strategies but whose treatment automatically allows a return to the former state (Guex 1986b).

Cancer pain is complex, for it involves acute and chronic elements at the same time. In the early stages, pain may be only acute, and treatment will relieve it. It is possibly the same with recurrences, correctly treated. But external factors may intervene. If for a particular patient, for example, the first signs of the disease were pain, then all subsequent pain will mean a recurrence and will give rise to distress. Albeit unconsciously, to have pain will perhaps mean to benefit from increased attention.

For the cancer patient, pain almost always has a harmful connotation, whether near or far away in time, but cultural, personal, relational and cognitive elements (notably what the person has understood about his illness) certainly play a part in it. Certain studies (Pilowsky and Spence 1976) have shown that anxiety, anger, sadness and depression can lower the threshold of pain. Similarly, these states induce overinterpretation of the body's messages, being out of proportion with the triggering organic factor. It is necessary for the doctor to have a comprehensive understanding of these phenomena and endeavour to intervene adequately.

It is clear that the growth of tumours offers a variety of physiological causes of pain. One only has to think of bony metastases, of the compression of internal organs, or the invasion of neural plexuses. Pain (caused by scarring) can also follow surgical mutilations or radiotherapy. If there is insufficient correlation between the pain and the extent of invasion of the tissues, one should consider the multidimensionality of the pain (Melzack *et al.* 1985), with its sensory factors (physiology), affective factors (individual emotional response) and cognitive factors (perception of pain and the capacity to respond to it).

This multifaceted approach is at the root of multidisciplinary consultations on the subject of pain, which integrate the opinion of various specialists, whether oncologists, psychiatrists, neurologists, neurosurgeons or anaesthetists. The patient must benefit from satisfactory relief in order to accept his diagnosis and the methods envisaged for his treatment. For patients with advanced disease, pain control must be sufficiently effective to enable them to live in the best possible condition and to die in comfort.

To clarify matters, Foley (1985) has established the broad categories of patients with pain which one meets with in the field of cancer medicine. They are:
– patients with acute cancer-related pain:
  (a) associated with the diagnosis of cancer;
  (b) associated with cancer therapy (surgery, chemotherapy or radiation);
– patients with chronic cancer-related pain:
  (a) associated with cancer progression;
  (b) associated with cancer therapy (surgery, chemotherapy or radiation);

- patients with pre-existing chronic pain and cancer-related pain;
- patients with a history of drug addiction and cancer-related pain:
  - (a) actively involved in illicit drug use;
  - (b) in methadone maintenance programmes;
  - (c) with a history of drug abuse; and
- dying patients with cancer-related pain.

Acute and chronic pain differ in their central modulation as well as in their clinical and therapeutic treatment. The experience of pain is subjective, and the doctor seldom has many ways to make an objective evaluation of it. It is best always to believe the patient. The clinical picture of acute pain is generally clear (except in elderly patients, where the problem may be complex) for it triggers a stimulation of the autonomic nervous system, and there is a fairly exact correlation between the patient's complaints and the results of physical examination (Spiegel and Bloom 1983). For chronic pain it is more difficult, since there is an adaptation of the autonomic nervous system which goes hand in hand with changes in personality, life-style, and function. Psychological symptoms are then predominant, notably problems with sleep, eating, and concentration, irritability, and other signs indicating a state of depression. This can be found in 25 per cent of the consulting population (Sternbach 1974). I will not return to the group of patients presenting with chronic pain before contracting cancer, except to say that one should not use what one knows of their case history as an excuse for complacency, for they are at grave risk of being the subject of errors in clinical interpretation and of serious difficulties in adaptation, disproportionate to their actual handicap. For those who present with substance abuse or drug dependency, as well as those who have been cured of addiction, one must understand that the psychological stress associated with the discovery of the disease puts them at great risk of relapse. One should show tolerance and avoid a judgemental attitude. Equally, one should expect to adapt the dose of analgesics and psychotropics, since these are people who will need higher doses to obtain relief (Futz and Senay 1975).

For the last group, that of terminal patients, the main concern should be to make the person comfortable. At this stage, analgesics should not be restricted, for it is no longer a matter of pharmacological theory but a search for effectiveness. To allow someone to die in great pain is not only terrible for the patient himself, but extremely distressing for the family and demoralizing for the medical team. The essential thing is to know how to understand the needs of the patient and to respond to them (Saunders 1982; American College of Physicians 1983).

It is recognized that a certain number of neurophysiological and neuropharmacological mechanisms intervene in the bones, the soft tissues, the lymphatic and blood vessels, the nerves and the viscera, activating and sensitizing the nocireceptors and the mechano-receptors by direct effect (compression or infiltration) or neuro-humoral means. Acute pain, either intermittent or continuous, may result. Generally, classic therapeutic measures are effective in controlling this type of pain. On the other hand, lesions or nerve sections, or plexual infiltrations, may produce partial damage to the nerve endings and membranes which will then be extremely sensitive to every new onslaught of the disease. After a certain time, nerve lesions give rise to deafferentation pains (i.e., pains produced by the neurone itself) through the hyperactivity of the central neurones, in the spinal cord and the thalamus.

To sum up, about 60 per cent of pain is caused directly by the tumour, 20 per cent is the result of treatment, and 20 per cent is independent of the cancer or its treatment and probably associated with individual factors (Foley 1982).

THE TREATMENT OF PAIN

The interventions available for controlling cancer pain may be classified into six groups: the minor, major, and adjuvant analgesics, neurosurgical and anaesthetic techniques, and the behavioural approach. All systemic analgesics act by inhibiting the perception of pain at the thalamic level, at the level of thalamic efferents towards the cerebral cortex, or on the pathways of thalamo-cortical and spino-cortical projection (Bonica 1979; Peters 1981; Foley 1982; Kocher 1982).

Minor analgesics (non-steroidal anti-inflammatory drugs)

These are the products of first choice for the treatment of moderate pain (Table 4.1). When the pain is severe, these are the means of potentiating narcotic analgesics. Aspirin, paracetamol, indomethacin, the derivatives of phenazone and mefenamic acid are effective within certain limits. Their long-term usage poses gastro-intestinal and haematological problems; on the other hand, they do not involve any physical tolerance or dependence. Their use is more beneficial for musculo-skeletal pain than for visceral pain. It is thought that they may act on the transmission of the pain impulse towards the spinal ganglia by way of the C and delta A fibres (Peters 1981).

Major analgesics (narcotics)

Here we distinguish among three main groups: derivatives of morphine, of pethidine [meperidine], and of methadone (Table 4.2). These are agonist and antagonist according to their capacity to bind themselves to opioid receptors. Morphine, traditionally administered by injection, is typically an agonist drug. It is now available in the form of a sustained-release tablet (MST Continus). The antagonist narcotics inhibit the effect of morphine on its receptors. Among them, there are medications which have analgesic properties and which are a mixture of agonist/antagonist. They have a limited application, for they produce psychomimetic effects in increased doses and, except for pentazocine, cannot be administered by drip. The best of them is buprenorphine, which has fewer side-effects and which leads to less dependence than morphine. Use of narcotic analgesics requires caution because of the tolerance and physical dependence to which they give rise. Tolerance implies that increased doses need to be used to maintain the same analgesic effect. Physical dependence is characterized by acute withdrawal symptoms. Psychological dependence, called 'addiction', is independent of physical dependence and of tolerance and is an acquired behaviour characteristic of drug addicts, whose manifestations are abuse and an active struggle to obtain the necessary substances. Because of a confusion between physical dependence and addiction – that is, psychological dependence – the administration of narcotic analgesics has often been inadequate for patients suffering from acute or chronic pain. The discovery of the role of the endorphins in the modulation of pain will perhaps now favour a re-evaluation of this attitude. The work done in British hospices shows that the prolonged use of these drugs with cancer patients and with other patients suffering from serious disease leads only to tolerance and physical dependence, but rarely to addiction (Porter and Jick 1980). In all cases, physical dependence is dissociated from psychological dependence. The American Medical Association (1980) and the American

College of Physicians (1983) have specified the use of these drugs in the treatment of the severe chronic pain which is associated with terminal illness. They defend the position of adequate pain control (that is to say, with the necessary doses of analgesics) so that the terminal patient can be without suffering. They have also underlined the need to educate doctors and other health professionals in the care of the cancer patient and the use of narcotic analgesics. One may sum up their proposals in the following way:

- Begin with a specific drug for a specific type of pain.
- Know the pharmacological effect of the drug prescribed, including:
     (a) the duration of the analgesic effect;
     (b) the pharmaco-kinetic properties of the drug; and
     (c) the equianalgesic properties of the drug and its route of administration.
- Adjust the type of administration to the needs of the patient.
- Administer the analgesic in a regular manner after initial measurement of its concentration in the blood. (Avoid the system of dosing on demand.)
- Use associated medication to produce supplementary analgesia and reduce side-effects (for example, non-steroidal anti-inflammatory drugs, antihistamines and amphetamines).
- Avoid associated medication that aggravates sedation without increasing analgesia, for example the benzodiazepines and the phenothiazines.
- Anticipate and treat side-effects, including:
     (a) sedation;
     (b) respiratory distress;
     (c) nausea, vomiting; and
     (d) constipation.
- Watch for the development of tolerance:
     (a) have in mind alternative narcotic analgesics; and
     (b) begin with half an equianalgesic dose and assess the blood concentration which brings relief of pain.
- Avoid acute withdrawal symptoms:
     (a) reduce the dose slowly;
     (b) use a diluted dose of naloxone (0.4 mg in 10 ml of saline solution) to correct respiratory depression in a physically dependent patient, and administer with care.
- Do not use placebos to ascertain the nature of the pain.
- Anticipate complications, and treat them, including:

(a) overdose;
(b) myoclonic seizures; and
(c) convulsions.

As a general rule, one cannot say that there are analgesic agents of choice, but rather a series of products which have been used effectively for treating cancer pain (Foley 1982). Morphine by mouth is the most common, but its use is still restricted in some states. Certain patients do not tolerate it well, and so one must employ alternative drugs, such as methadone, a very active opioid taken orally which has a longer duration of action than morphine, and the little known oxycodone. Often inadequate doses are given, and in going from one treatment to another, insufficient account is taken of analgesic equivalents (called 'equianalgesic properties'). Moreover, one should always be able to administer a medication according to its plasma half-life, in regular doses, calculated on the duration of the analgesic effect. The pharmacological plasma level must be maintained above the minimum effective concentration to be efficacious. So, the time necessary to find a balance, after several doses, is variable for each analgesic drug: twenty-four hours for morphine, or five to seven days for methadone. Certain combinations are effective: a narcotic and a non-narcotic (such as aspirin or ibuprofen), a narcotic and an antihistamine (promethazine) or more rarely an amphetamine. 'Brompton Cocktail', formerly used in Great Britain, was composed of heroin or morphine, cocaine, phenothiazine, alcohol, and chloroform, and was found to be effective for 90 per cent of terminal patients. However, Twycross and Lack (1984) showed that analgesic effectiveness was due to the presence of the narcotic, and for this reason proposed to avoid such cocktails, suggesting that cocaine should be omitted and that heroin should always be replaced by morphine. According to Mount et al. (1976), liquid morphine in a 10 per cent solution of alcohol is very well tolerated.

The routes of administration must also be adapted to the needs of the patients. The oral route is, of course, the most practical, but depending on how well the substance is absorbed, it may prove to be ineffective. Use of the syringe-driver has now revolutionized the local administration of certain drugs, since the patient himself has autonomy and can control the dose to achieve effective pain relief at all times.

Adjuvant analgesics

Adjuvant analgesics constitute a third group of products, such as the anticonvulsants, the phenothiazines, the butyrophenones, the tricyclic antidepressants, the antihistamines, the amphetamines, the steroids and the antiparkinsonism drugs. These products are analgesic in certain painful states, according to mechanisms not yet established. Their interest resides in the fact that they potentiate or block neurotransmitter function. Tricyclic antidepressants are effective in the depression brought about by severe pain and for the pain itself in increasing the level of available serotonin. Certain studies suggest that the cells which use serotonin form one of the pathways by which pain is controlled, which come from a part of the brain rich in endorphin cells, and end with cells that inhibit pain lower down on the spinal cord (Kocher 1982).

At present, I incline to the view that all these products are not as effective in the relief of pain as the analgesic narcotics, but may be combined with them.

The anaesthetic and neurosurgical approach

These techniques include neurostimulation, neuropharmacological injection, and neuroablative surgical techniques. The best established is transcutaneous electrical nerve stimulation (TENS) (Long and Hagfors 1975). There is also direct medullary and thalamic stimulation.

The injection of local anaesthetics or neurolytic agents is the current practice and may be given on an outpatient basis, particularly in the case of sympathetic blockade (Løfstrøm 1969; Long and Hagfors 1975). The infusion of anaesthetics and opiates into the epidural and intrathecal space has more limited indications. Neurosurgical operations are highly specialized and are reserved for exceptional situations that require precise evaluation of the nature of the pain, the prognosis of the patient and his understanding of the potential risks as against the expected benefit (Fankhauser 1986).

The behavioural approach

Cognitive-behavioural methods include relaxation, biofeedback, desensitization and self-hypnosis. They will be dealt with in Chapter 12. The principal aim of these interventions is to allow the patient himself to be active in the management of his illness, to gain a feeling of control over events and to fight effectively against his feeling of despair and abandonment. This puts at the disposal of patients a certain number of ways in which they can regain mastery of themselves, develop strategies for adapting to pain, and facilitate their tolerance of treatment and of all the subjective and negative symptoms brought about by the disease (Redd *et al.* 1982a).

Table 4.1 Minor and major analgesics for weak to moderate pain

	Equianalgesic dose* (mg)	Duration of action (hrs)	Plasma half-life (hrs)
Aspirin	650	4–6	3–5
Paracetamol [Acetaminophen]	650	4–6	1–4
Codeine	32	4–6	3
Dextropropoxyphene	65	4–6	12
Pentazocine	30	4–6	2–3

* Theoretical strength of the medication, in comparison with that of aspirin. These doses do not represent actual tablets.

Table 4.2 Major analgesics for severe pain

Agonist narcotics	Adminis-tration	Equianalgesic dose* (mg)	Duration of action (hrs)	Plasma half-life (hrs)
Morphine	IM (intramuscular)	10	4–6	2–3–5
	PO (by mouth)	60	4–7	2–3–5
Methadone	IM	10	6	15–30
	PO	20	6	15–30
Agonist-antagonists				
Pentazocine	IM	60	4–6	2–3
	PO	180	4–7	2–3
Partial agonists				
Buprenorphine	IM	0.4	4–6	?
	SL (sublingual)	0.8	5–6	?

* Based on single intramuscular doses in comparison with the relative power of morphine. The recommended starting dose by mouth is 30 mg for morphine, 5 mg for methadone.

Chapter 5

Psychopharmacology and cancer

There is no general rule that allows one to choose a psychotropic drug that is truly adapted to a specific situation. This is particularly the case in cancer medicine, where until now no psychopharmacological research has studied the special needs of cancer patients. This is an omission, for cancer, as we have seen, is a condition where psychological distress is frequent (Holland 1977; Derogatis 1982: Table 5.1).

Clinicians tend to prescribe medications which they know and which they have found useful in their practice (Table 5.2).

Derogatis *et al.* (1979b) analysed 1,579 admissions in three cancer outpatient centres. They discovered that half the patients were taking one or more psychotropic drugs, 44 per cent for sleep disorders, 25 per cent for nausea and vomiting, 17 per cent for emotional problems, and the rest for pain, convulsions, or in anticipation of particular medical procedures (biopsies, insertion of cannulae, etc.).

There are four broad categories of prescribed drugs: the hypnosedatives, the anxiolytics, the antipsychotics and the antidepressants. This last category is sometimes misused, since people have difficulty in detecting depression correctly, even though it is common among cancer patients (Greenblatt *et al.* 1975; Ward *et al.* 1979).

HYPNOSEDATIVES AND ANXIOLYTICS

These represent 70 per cent of all prescriptions. They are primarily the benzodiazepines, to which the risk of addiction has been recently emphasized. They are nevertheless the products of choice for quickly calming excessive distress and ensuring correct sedation. For sleep disorders, temazepam, lorazepam and, in Europe, flunitrazepam are the most common. For anxiolysis, lorazepam is used in the United

States and Britain; in other European countries, the preference is for bromazepam and clorazepate dipotassium.

One must watch out for not uncommon adverse effects such as drowsiness, asthenia, or ataxia and disorders of memory and concentration among elderly people. Paradoxical reactions (hyperexcitation, hallucinations, muscular hypertonicity) have been reported, as well as withdrawal syndromes among subjects taking high doses over long periods.

ANTIPSYCHOTICS (NEUROLEPTICS)

For the most part, these are phenothiazine derivatives (chlorpromazine, methotrimeprazine, thioridazine), the butyrophenones (haloperidol) and the thioxanthenes (chlorprothixene).

In situations where the patient is distressed because he feels his body is being invaded by the tumour, this particular type of anguish may be relieved by low doses of neuroleptics. For example, haloperidol, in very low doses (0.5 mg or 1 mg three times a day), has an anxiolytic effect, with little risk of extrapyramidal symptoms. In a cancer patient it is never necessary to exceed these doses, except in the presence of psychotic symptoms. Methotrimeprazine and thioridazine may be prescribed at night in one dose of 25 mg or more, adapted to the patient according to his symptomatology, his height and his weight.

Neuroleptics, of which chlorpromazine has been the leader, are medications which are effective for generalized anxiety, nausea and vomiting, and sometimes for exogenous psychoses (toxic or organic). They are anticholinergic and antihistaminic, inhibit the action of serotonin and dopamine, block peripheral adrenergic receptors, and reduce peripheral input into the reticular system, which produces sedation. In high doses they depress the activity of the brain-stem and stimulate the extrapyramidal system. Their absorption is rapid, since the action appears in thirty minutes and continues for about four hours. Sixty to seventy per cent of the substance is metabolized in the liver; small quantities are eliminated in the urine. These drugs should therefore be administered with caution in the presence of liver dysfunction.

In medium doses, the principal indications are as follows:

– the suppression of nausea and vomiting such as occur during the course of radiotherapy, chemotherapy, uraemia, and terminal illness;

- pruritus, particularly that associated with neurodermatitis (they have less effect on the pruritus accompanying jaundice and the lymphomas); and
- the potentiation of the effects of sedative and analgesic medication: the addition of a neuroleptic allows a reduction of around 30 per cent in the dosage of opiates.

Neuroleptics, in moderate or low doses, are well tolerated. The main side-effects are:

- Hypotension, involving an inhibition of the central pressor reflexes, a sympathetic peripheral blockage and sometimes a diminution of myocardial function.
- Extrapyramidal symptoms. The Parkinsonian syndrome, which can also be observed with the administration of metoclopramide (commonly used by general practitioners in Europe), should be controlled by anticholinergics such as procyclidine. Reduction of dose usually leads to the disappearance of the symptoms. Dyskinetic manifestations can be very severe (stiff neck, opisthotonos, dysarthria, involuntary muscular movements such as spasm of the tongue and oculogyric crises). These reactions are calmed very quickly by the intramuscular injection of procyclidine.
- Cholestatic jaundice is rare, as are haematological symptoms such as leucopenia, eosinophilia or agranulocytosis.

Since nausea and vomiting are often the result of conditioning, it is difficult to allay them with a single medication. The standard anti-

Table 5.1 Distribution of prescription of psychotropic drugs in oncology (after Derogatis 1982)

Reason for prescribing	Overall (%)	Anxio-lytic (%)	Antipsy-chotic (%)	Antide-pressant (%)	Hypno-sedative (%)
Psychological distress	17	57	8	71	1
Sleep disorders	44	7	1	23	85
Nausea and vomiting	25	6	90	0	1
Anticipation of particular medical procedures	12	22	0	0	14
Pain	1	4	1	6	0
Seizure	1	4	0	0	0

Table 5.2 Proportions of the different psychotropic drugs most commonly used in oncology for each category of disorder

Anxiolytics (%)	Antipsychotics (%)	Antidepressants (%)	Hypnosedatives (%)
Diazepam/ Bromazepam (74)	Methotrimeprazine (83)	Amitriptyline (75)	Flurazepam/ Flunitrazepam (71)
Phenobarbitone (8)	Chlorpromazine (11)	Imipramine (15)	Pentobarbitone/ Phenobarbitone (19)
Hydroxyzine (8)	Thioridazine (2)	Clomipramine (5)	Chloral derivatives (9)
Chlordiazepoxide (6)	Haloperidol (2)	Doxepin (5)	
Oxazepam/Lorazepam (2)			

emetics are the phenothiazines and the butyrophenones. But the use of lorazepam and domperidone as suppositories has had good results.

ANTIDEPRESSANTS

A disease as threatening as cancer often induces a depressive mood. It could be said that this is a normal reaction, adapted to the situation, and that a certain level of distress, of dysphoria, or of grief plays a part in adaptive mechanisms. Such patients can often be helped to feel better simply by emotional support and psychological counselling: they should not be prescribed antidepressants automatically. However, if the depressive mood persists, gets worse, or impedes the principal treatment, one should not be afraid of prescribing antidepressants.

These medicines should be administered to begin with in low doses for a week, then increased progressively until an effective therapeutic threshold has been reached. Generally, the symptoms of depression improve progressively and according to their order of appearance – for example lack of appetite or retardation. Care should be taken here, for people who are suddenly more active and less slowed up may retain depressive ideation – a critical moment for the appearance of suicidal ideas.

The commonest and most effective antidepressants are the tricyclic drugs. For these, the initial dose is usually from 50 to 75 mg daily, either divided into three or given in a single dose at night. The tricyclic antidepressants, among which imipramine and amitriptyline have been the leaders, have an action which is either serotoninergic or adrenergic. Their full effect is generally not felt for two to three weeks; their length of action is short – there is no long-term accumulation. They rarely potentiate other commonly prescribed medicines, except pain relievers (Table 5.3).

Once the optimum dose has been settled (between 50 and 100 mg daily), the main problem is to control side-effects (Table 5.4). No improvement after three to six weeks indicates that, in the therapeutic alliance between doctor and patient, either the essential role of psychological support or that of medication has not been clearly established. If a more biological standpoint is taken, this is also the sign that the patient is resistant to the type of product used. The treatment must then be changed and another antidepressant substituted, with a different neurotransmitter effect. Thus a serotoninergic (clomipramine, imipramine) should be replaced by a noradrenergic (nortriptyline, desipramine).

Side-effects are a frequent cause of refusal of treatment on the part of patients. Generally, patients will accept side-effects and put up with them if they are well informed and see that their doctors know about them and keep them under control. The tricyclics constitute the first generation of these products; they are effective for all kinds of depression, above all if there are problems of eating, sleeping, and a diurnal variation of mood, with morning deterioration.

The tertiary amines (imipramine, amitriptyline) are the drugs of choice, even though they have more intense anticholinergic effects than the secondary amines (desipramine, nortriptyline). The tertiary amines are, in fact, more powerful in blocking the re-uptake of serotonin than are the secondary amines, which is a pharmacological advantage. The second category has a mixed serotoninergic and adrenergic activity (above all by the intermediary of the metabolites).

The sedative effect of clomipramine, doxepin, and amitriptyline, usually considered to be unpleasant, may be appropriately used in states of distress, and particularly at night, so that it is not necessary to add a sedative.

Table 5.3 Intensity of the inhibition of re-uptake of neurotransmitters

Drugs	5HT Serotonin	NA Noradrenaline	DA Dopamine
Clomipramine	+ + + +	0	0
Amitriptyline	+ + +	+	0
Imipramine	+ + +	+ +	0
Nortriptyline	+ +	+ + +	0
Desipramine	0	+ + + +	0

Table 5.4 Side-effects of the tricyclics and their treatment

Cardio-vascular

Characteristics	Signs and symptoms	Treatment
These symptoms result from: – alpha blockage – negative inotropic effects	Orthostatic hypotension	Around 20% of patients complain of dizziness; they must be taught to stand up in two movements.
– anticholinergic effects	Changes in ECG: prolongation of the QT segment; depression of the ST segment; flattening of the T wave	These changes are reversible and of little clinical significance. For patients suffering conduction problems, tricyclics should be avoided.

Endocrine system

Characteristics	Signs and symptoms	Treatment
The symptoms are the result of the effects of the drugs on the diencephalon.	Weight gain	(This may result from the hypothalamic effect or from an improvement in appetite which follows the remission of symptoms.)

Table 5.4   cont.

Endocrine system (cont.)

Characteristics	Signs and symptoms	Treatment
	Amenorrhoea and galactorrhoea	Patients are not disturbed by amenorrhoea as long as one explains to them that it is temporary.
	Loss of libido and impotence	Will improve with the lifting of the depression or the stopping of medication

Autonomic nervous system

Characteristics	Signs and symptoms	Treatment
The symptoms seem to result from the anticholinergic effect.	Dry mouth	Eat chewing-gum or use a mouthwash.
	Constipation	Monitor bowel activity; give dietary advice and/or laxatives.
The symptoms seem to depend on the dose.	Blurred vision	Disappears with time. If there is ocular pain, watch out for narrow-angle glaucoma.
The symptoms disappear with the development of tolerance.	Urinary problems	Avoid these products in prostatic cases.
	Vasomotor problems	Sweating and hot flushes: patients should be reassured that these symptoms are transitory.

Table 5.4   cont.

Allergic, blood, hepatic and cutaneous effects

Characteristics	Signs and symptoms	Treatment
A family or personal history of allergy is a contra-indication to the administration of tricyclics.	Cholestasis, jaundice	Monitor alkaline phosphatase.
	Agranulocytosis	Watch the blood count.
	Urticaria and photosensitivity	The presence of skin disorders necessitates cessation of treatment.
	Increase of transaminases	Monitor hepatic function.

Central nervous system

Characteristics	Signs and symptoms	Treatment
The symptoms result principally from the anticholinergic effect, active at the cortical as well as the subcortical level.	Slight tremor	Interruption of treatment or complementary administration of betablockers
	Dysarthria and ataxia	Sign of too high drug dosage
	Rarely, hyperactivity, disorientation, memory disorders	Interruption of treatment
	State of dreamlike confusion	Interruption of treatment, especially in the elderly

Chapter 6
The diagnosis

GENERAL

Cancer is a sequence of events linked one with another, which begins with the first signs of the disease, continues with treatments, hospitalizations, convalescence, and remission, and ends, possibly, with recurrence and death. The diagnosis is at the head of this long chain. The way in which it is communicated will bring with it, in the patient and his family, reactions that will determine the whole course of the disease. Emotional adaptation begins on the day of the diagnosis.

In the present context of specialization, it is possible that the doctor in charge of treatment will not be the same as the one who gave the diagnosis of cancer. This is the whole difficulty of the general practitioner's intervention: he will perhaps have given the initial information and will be personally committed to a relationship of trust, while knowing that he will not be taking on the entire care of the case. He will often have to send his patient to a specialist colleague, whom he will be careful to present as a significant and competent source of support. The specialist, for his part, should also be personally committed, without ignoring the pre-existing network and the other contributors.

Whether general practitioner or specialist, the doctor will encourage adaptation to the disease by giving adequate replies and detailed information. One must avoid pretences, which fuel anxiety, distress and depressive reactions (Schneider 1969a). It is not a question of making the patient completely dependent, but of establishing the moments of least resistance, to offer supplementary help. The time of diagnosis is therefore very favourable for this (Morgan and Engel 1969; Dufey *et al.* 1980).

THE TRUTH

For a long time, the custom was to reduce information to the patient as much as possible, putting him in the picture only in a very general way. Up until the 1970s, the preference was for not telling the patient the truth (McIntosh 1974). A common practice was to tell the members of the family, who then decided among themselves whether the patient was able to take the diagnosis (Fitts and Ravdin 1953). This involved a system of double accountability, between what the therapeutic team and the families thought and said. The most interesting thing is that this duality also formed part of the adaptive mechanisms of the patient, who had played his part by not revealing what he had understood on his own. Each one thought, therefore, that he was protecting the other in the best way, but that gave rise to serious problems of misunderstanding, which could finally lead to a breakdown of communication. At all events, the non-access to sources of elementary information leads the patient to do his own research, to create for himself his own picture of the situation, and to imagine the worst. This is a factor that aggravates distress and depressive states. In the final stage, it may lead to a syndrome of sensory deprivation, either delirium or a state of unreality, when contact with the outside world is no longer guaranteed or experienced as reliable. This kind of attitude has changed, in principle, in recent years (Novack et al. 1979).

An enquiry has shown that 98 per cent of American doctors now prefer the truth (Oken 1961; Friedman 1970). The patients share this view, reckoning that it is their right not to be left in ignorance and to know what to expect, so as to be able to share in decision-making and put their affairs in order (McIntosh 1974).

In announcing the diagnosis, the doctor must know what to say and how to say it; how to observe, listen, interpret and better understand the wishes and needs of the patient; how to present his treatment plan and how to defend it. This approach will be facilitated if he knows in which psychosocial context the patient belongs, where he comes from, and which health professionals he has already had occasion to meet as regards his illness.

The aspects the doctor should look out for may be summed up as follows:

- what the patient already knows of the disease;
- what conclusion he has already been able to draw (including any misapprehensions he has acquired);

- the nature of his family structure (so as to identify the family member or friend who is the most important to him);
- what type of social and familial milieu he belongs to (to determine his capacity for trusting the doctor, and how he is accustomed to express his emotions in stressful situations); and
- his age, his intelligence, his wish to understand, and his emotional stability.

THE INTERVIEW WITH THE PATIENT

The interview should not be hurried. There must be time to introduce things conscientiously and calmly and so that the patient has the opportunity to understand and to ask questions. The interview should take place in privacy, in such a way that he can express his real feelings without embarrassment. If he wishes, the patient can be accompanied by the partner or the closest family members, who can be reassuring and bring another point of view to bear on the matter. But this practice should not be instituted automatically: one should try to avoid infantilization and dependence.

Language should be adapted as well, avoiding terms which are too abstract, superfluous, or scientific. If possible, adopt the terms appropriate to the person one is dealing with, and be aware of his system of terminology. One knows that for certain people, for example, to have a cannula inserted means that there is fluid somewhere, and the thought of fluid sometimes brings thoughts of the end; whereas perhaps the doctor simply has in mind a needle biopsy or marrow puncture (Boltanski 1971).

It is not a question of modifying or denying the truth, but of deciding which aspects of the truth are the most helpful or will be the least wounding for the patient. Intuitively, one must know how to distinguish between the truth and the whole truth (Saunders 1982). The doctor should proceed by small steps, honestly. One must not forget the defence mechanisms, which at each moment may block the receptive capacity of the patient. He will perhaps indicate himself, by his expression or his posture (his nonverbal language), the amount of information he expects and can deal with. Long silences, or the avoidance of direct eye contact, may mean that he has reached the limit of the tolerable or the threshold of what he can take in. This is variable: certain patients will say that they wish to know absolutely everything, while others will declare clearly that they don't want to hear anything.

It is absolutely essential to give hope that the treatment that they will receive will work, and one must believe this oneself. False reassurances are counter-productive and may erode trust in the doctor. One way of working is to explain exactly what is going to happen, and the remission which one can thereby expect, while still anticipating future stages and speaking of other possible treatments. Finally, patients and family members must be encouraged to ask questions. One must say that one will always be available to review all the issues, when they have had the time to think them over, and to reply to any new questions, according to the various stages. At all events, one must insist on the fact that one will stay by their side whatever happens (Bertakis 1977; Ahrens 1979).

THE PATIENT

To communicate a diagnosis, which is still a shock and an existential blow, great skill is required. Many patients will say later, even if the thing has been well done, that they were shocked, terrified, panic-stricken or shattered. Most of their initial reactions will serve to protect them, offering them the time and space to adapt themselves. These are the moments favouring denial, which the doctor must understand and prepare himself to face. Without denial, distress might be too overwhelming and create an intolerable state of crisis. For some people, moreover, simply hearing the word 'cancer' means a mental block and total incapacity to understand anything that follows. One must not be afraid of repeating things several times (Siegrist 1976).

Carers must be prepared for these moments of extreme emotion in their patients. We have seen reactions of rage, of aggression, of violent hostility. Anxiety may show itself by tears and uncontrolled crying. Depression is a common symptom, which should be seen as a normal emotional reaction. Too often, and one has seen this in the psychodynamic of people with cancer, the patient reacts only too little, given his long experience of emotional repression.

We must speak here of the problem of guilt. For many, guilt seems to come from a common impression that cancer is 'shameful', a sign of disgrace. Patients will have the tendency to blame themselves and to look for the causes of this misfortune in their past behaviour or their way of life. They may also attribute the responsibility for it to the external world, to the decadence of society, nuclear energy, the attitude of their relations, or the doctors who have not been any use.

These feelings, perhaps irrational, are extremely common, and one must know about them to be able to respond to them. It is sometimes helpful to be able to state right away that there is no obvious causal relationship between the kind of life the patient has led, the person he is, and cancer – a disease that can strike anybody.

Chapter 7

The doctor

THE DOCTOR–PATIENT RELATIONSHIP

In Greek mythology, the role of the 'death-dodger' character was taken by Sisyphus. Jealous Zeus had sent him Thanatos (Death), but the wily Greek managed to entice him and take him prisoner. The god of gods then had to send an emissary to deliver Death and thus avoid for humanity the appalling catastrophe that nobody could die any more!

Later this myth was to include the character of the 'death-dodger' doctor, who could not really begin to provide effective rational and scientific methods until the end of the nineteenth century (after the discoveries of Louis Pasteur and Claude Bernard).

In former ages, the doctor could only fulfil his role of relieving pain or delaying death in a very modest way. Now he feels better equipped in a certain number of fields and he has adopted the habit, as often as he can, of banishing from his mind the possible proximity of death – except perhaps in cancer medicine, where he is put into a difficult and ambiguous situation like no other (Schneider 1980).

If he only puts faith in the extraordinary progress which has been made in the biological field of cancer, and concentrates on the re-establishment of health and on survival, he is quickly disabused by bitter therapeutic setbacks and recurrences, indeed the death of his patients. If, on the other hand, he allows himself to be contaminated by the pessimism of his intuition and his personal experiences, he is then surprised by the success of certain therapeutic methods, the length of remissions, and the spectacular cures.

To look after a cancer patient is an uncertain and somewhat contradictory enterprise. There are two aspects which tend to come to the fore: on the one hand, what one thinks about cancer as a human being, with the series of emotional reactions, feelings of power-lessness and of fear which accompany it; on the other hand, what one must believe in and what one must undertake, by reason of one's responsibility and the scientific resources which must be put at the patient's disposal.

I stress this ambivalence to give voice to the oncologists, who say that faced with certain treatments or with certain interventions, they sometimes have a good mind to give up fighting for their patients. The task is indeed very difficult: one must always think of the patient, while taking account of all the aspects which are touched on in the other chapters of this book.

The diagnosis marks the start of the doctor–patient relationship. Many patients see their doctor, with his qualifications and experience, as the principal source of help when faced with illness. He must offer a buffer against confusion, despair and fear, while showing himself to be effective, in his words and gestures, and moreover empathic (Sapir 1980; Pierloot 1983). The patient needs to be sure that the doctor is competent and committed to his interests, and that he takes account of the difficult experience that he is undergoing.

The doctor must show his commitment, confidence and understanding during the whole course of the case. No one is better able than he to explain to the patient the therapeutic plan and its benefits and risks; to know what to say and what amount of information to give, in an atmosphere of truthfulness but with tact, and choosing the right moment in relation to what the patient asks and what he can take in. The tone is given by the doctor's own personality, by his beliefs, his training, his clinical experience, and also the kind of relationship that he has built up with the patient. In a word, one must know how to respond to the expectation of the person one is treating, and one must respect his role in decisions which concern him, with good listening skills and with tolerance. But one should not let him get too much in the way of medical efficiency, which is conditioned more and more by the stringency of therapeutic protocols conceived elsewhere (Sapir 1973; Schneider 1978, 1980).

While taking account of all these factors, the doctor–patient relationship in cancer medicine will constantly alternate between various models, according to Schneider's (1976) definitions:

– *The scientific relationship.* This is the closest to that of the model of medical studies, when one examines the body and the organs and compares the results of the different clinical and para-clinical tests. This type of relationship must last for the time which is essential for the investigation, and thereafter for periods in the course of consultations, the time necessary to follow the evolution of the disease, to know where one is and to omit nothing. This scientific relationship is the attitude of the doctor who wants to know what he is doing, but who is considering primarily the disease and not the patient in his overall view.

– *The maintenance relationship* (also called 'chronic relationship'). When a treatment is under way and lasts several weeks, even several months, the consultations then take place in a fairly stereotyped way. The patient knows that he must go to have a blood test and an X-ray before going to see his doctor. If there is no new clinical element, he will be asked about two or three things which are always the same: his weight, the side-effects of the treatment, his general quality of life, but without going into detail. This relationship implies a lesser submission of the patient, who little by little, in his own way, becomes a specialist in his own disease and knows more or less how he should ask for help, especially when certain problems arise.

The maintenance relationship often corresponds with a period of calm and 'perfect accord' between patient and doctor for, apparently in any case, each one knows where he is. We must beware, nevertheless, lest this relationship also corresponds to a certain 'chronic' adjustment of both doctor's and patient's defences. Both of them have calmed their distress and their insecurity and have made a temporary pact not to disturb anything in their relationship. This does not exclude the possibility that the patient may all the same pass through serious times of doubt or fear, but he will not bring it up if he is not encouraged to do so.

– *The relationship of help and support.* Schneider (1976) makes a distinction between these two kinds of relationship. According to him, help implies a hierarchical relationship between the one who wants to help, and finds a certain satisfaction in it, and the one who is helped. The latter must admit his needs, his weakness, or his incompetence. The doctor takes a certain number of initiatives on behalf of the patient and knows what is good for him. This is a classical type of psychosocial approach when the patient is still at home but already at an advanced stage of his disease, and when he expects that difficulties will be smoothed out for him (social services, transport, supplementary aids such as a hospital bed for home use, for example).

The supportive relationship is of another kind. It implies that the patient himself asks for special psychological help, independently of the technical measures which may be put in hand. Here the doctor guides the patient's footsteps while providing help and comfort. The doctor thus puts himself partly in the patient's shoes, but he does not entirely take his place, and allows him control of the situation. It is a matter of empowering the patient by boosting his self-worth and self-esteem, thus increasing his psychological resistance to the disease by giving reassurance and a feeling of security.

– *The subjective interpersonal relationship*. This is a more advanced and developed stage of relationship, which appears following on from an implicit or explicit agreement between the doctor and his patient. There must have been a previous relationship of trust, where the doctor's attitude of listening and of benevolent neutrality encourages the patient to speak spontaneously of his feelings and concerns. According to Balint and Balint (1961), this is the 'flush' moment of attunement between two personalities, of a certain intensity, where the patient has the freedom to use the doctor as he wishes so as to introduce him into his drama. In this kind of interaction, the doctor may possibly allow himself to make certain observations to his patient and establish links with his unconscious psychological conflicts. He will do this without fear of wounding his self-esteem or of giving him the impression that he rejects him, because the patient himself will have shown that he was ready to listen. One might say that the subjective interpersonal relationship is *the relationship of quality* that one would wish to establish in oncology, for it offers a certain freedom with respect to the whole problem of cancer and tends to avoid the distressing ambiguities described above. In fact, it does involve a certain number of constraints and frustrations, or feelings of powerlessness in the face of the reality of the disease, without going so far as to interrupt therapy or giving the impression that there is no more to be done. The patient actually feels that the treatment is moving to a more existential level. He knows that he is valued and understood in his feelings and his personal history, independently of the purely medical history which belongs in his file.

THE TRAINING OF THE DOCTOR

Until recently, it was assumed that the young doctor should auto-matically possess the sensitivity and the psychological open-minded-ness necessary in the doctor–patient relationship and should be capable, from an innate knowledge, of confronting all situations, even the most distressing.

At the present time, training in medical psychology (psychosocial medicine) is much more developed and systematic. Unfortunately, too often it is those who already have a well-developed personal sensitivity who are interested in this aspect of the matter, rather than those who have need of it. Sapir (1984) calls this move a training no longer 'in order to' (as 'in order to' be a good technician) but the training 'by' ('by' meaning involving personal change, for a better relational approach). This is the opening up to the world of the emotions, attitudes and counter-attitudes which are experienced as much by the carer as by the cared-for. It is an encouragement to reflect on the importance of what is felt during the course of the disease and the treatment (Chardot 1984; Raimbault 1984; Schneider 1985).

This experience cannot be exclusively theoretical and is not reducible to a cognitive body of knowledge. The best method is practical experience, with broad exchanges with others and possibly with the method of case discussion in Balint groups (groups of practising doctors who regularly present the complex relational situations encountered with their patients, under the leadership of a psychiatrist).

We have seen in the chapter on diagnosis that most doctors seem ready now to confront their distress and are no longer afraid of facing the truth clearly and simply with their patients. But here, too, there are various steps.

Maguire (1984, 1985), having conducted an enquiry among general practitioners, has well demonstrated what one might call 'sins of omission'. 'Sinning by omission' is to say things only in reply to questions and without providing too much information spon-taneously. It is also to avoid part of the truth, often at the instigation of relatives who do not feel capable of facing the patient's distress. Such rules allow doctors to escape from the difficult task of establishing in a clear and well-founded way what the patient wants and is ready to know. In the short term, this certainly avoids many problems. For instance, one does not deny the difficulties, but encourages people to ask for additional information elsewhere, from more specialized colleagues or on their next hospital visit. The omission consists of avoiding finding out directly about the life of patients in relation to their progress and the treatment, unless they complain about them of their own accord. The excuse given by these doctors arises from the ambiguity mentioned above – that is to say that we know too little about the aetiology of cancer to be able to give explanations, or that treatments, notably chemotherapy for certain very resistant tumours or surgery for breast cancer, are too controversial from the scientific point of view. It is also that they are afraid of not being able to discuss matters clearly with the patient. To ask him automatically how he feels and how he is getting on always gives the impression that one is going to open up chasms of unspeakable anguish which are difficult to cope with. This is why some doctors consider that it is wiser to avoid dialogue and not run the risk of seeing the patient express very strong feelings of anger, anxiety, despair or guilt. How can these doctors channel such emotions and, above all, control the doubts which are growing in their minds? If they have not had the time to think about their own life, their own death and their own anguish, they will tend to run away from the guilt of not being able to control everything, of not having answers to every question.

Many doctors spend considerable energy in quite simply avoiding listening to people; it would sometimes be easier to face up to it, while knowing full well that at that precise moment no one could do any better. Happily, the most common attitude at present is to open up discussion, but it is clear that this is not the easiest route, for it implies a personal encounter.

THE DOCTOR'S EXPERIENCE

The exercise of listening means preparing oneself to analyse one's own reactions in the face of suffering and death. There is sometimes a risk here of being paralysed in one's therapeutic action, or on the other hand of tipping over into excessive interventionism as a way of channelling rising distress. But one can listen while also being aware of this.

In fact, carers are subjected to the same emotions and fears as their patients. They may lose heart, deny the truth, and avoid problems. At worst, these mechanisms risk isolating them completely from their patients. The capacity for helping may be completely undermined by their own feelings or their perception of things; this is the role of pessimism, as described above. This happens above all if the doctor or the care-giver over-identifies with his patient, if for example they are of the same age or have the same kind of interests, or if the patient reminds him of a relative. If he feels too inadequate or impotent, the doctor may also project his anger on to another, on the family – by keeping them out – or on the health-care team, which he will find inadequate. On the other hand, if he gets overwhelmingly involved, he may lose his indispensable clear-headedness.

To adopt a position of care-giver is to know how to be empathic while keeping a certain distance with regard to the patient and his disease. It is not a question of a distance which takes one away from the feeling and suffering of the other, but of an 'intellectual' distance which ensures objectivity and reduces the effects of a too-strong identification.

If distancing consists of coolness, it is no good. If generosity of contact leads to fusion, the effectiveness of the carer is lessened or nullified (Tyner 1985).

Faced with a patient who is not able to accept reality, or who denies the evidence, the doctor may become angry, which will then reinforce his guilt. At the moment when someone dies whom he has followed for long years, he may conceive the idea that he has failed in his task. On the other hand, a too-long agony may also lead him into anticipatory grief, which will push him towards shortening suffering according to his own perspective and without taking account of what may be the opinion of the patient or of his relatives.

To escape from this flood of contradictory feelings, some doctors retreat behind the façade of a meticulous treatment regime and spend as little time as possible with their patients, or they delegate this task to paramedical staff or psychiatrists.

Treating a cancer patient today demands a good deal of time, skill and sensitivity on the part of the practitioner but also of health-care teams. In fact, it is difficult to be the only one confronted by a disease which no longer demands merely technical or psychological competence but which also involves many ethical and sociological problems: death, pain, suffering, mutilation, isolation, media information, euthanasia, research, informed consent, determination to stay alive, and the risks of therapy. All these concepts should form an integral part of everyone's training.

The doctor should have other resources available to support his efforts, even if it is sometimes difficult to recognize his limits; this new concept of integrated care, involving teamwork, or close collaboration in the case of general practitioners and hospital centres, allows great possibilities for exchange of ideas and for ventilating tensions or sharing information. Nurses, social workers, clergy and psychiatrists can contribute effective complementary support and a starting-point for talking about psychosocial problems and finding solutions.

The doctor–patient relationship, but also the relationship between health-care team and patient in oncology, boils down finally not so much to a synthesis of precepts but to an attitude which might be termed 'ethical'. For the carer, it is not a matter of an interiorized constraint or an abstract imperative, or of an instinct absorbed from elsewhere, but rather of a moral conscience which arises from contact with the patient. The other person, the patient, by his simple presence and the tragedy which he is experiencing, forms a spontaneous resistance to our efforts, not frustrating them but calling them into question by throwing us back to the limit of our resources, 'our glorious living spontaneity', as Emmanuel Levinas puts it. This illustrates the huge difficulty of the doctor–patient relationship in oncology (Levinas 1982).

THE ROLE OF THE PSYCHIATRIST OR PSYCHOLOGIST

The psychiatrist is consulted first of all for psychological and emotional problems arising from the diagnosis, the progression of the illness, and the various treatments. This is primarily the case when anxious or depressive states are more severe than is generally tolerated by health-care teams, when these states do not respond to the usual drugs or when they last too long (Holland 1977; Maguire 1985). It is also usual when these states interfere with the smooth running of therapy and when patients refuse to communicate or oppose treatment that is planned. These problems push carers to the limits of their skill and seriously call into question their ability to influence or help the patient, which they find hard to cope with. This category includes the cognitive disorders caused by an organic cerebral lesion or by a psychotic reaction to the shock of the disease. The breakdown of communication which results compromises the usual consensus according to which being admitted into integrated care automatically implies acceptance of the help provided.

More generally, the psychiatrist is able to offer special focus on the emotional aspects of the illness and a more comprehensive understanding of the patient's needs, personality or background. This may help to improve the possibilities of a therapeutic partnership with the patient (Guex and Barrelet 1984).

These are not the only situations in which the psychiatrist can be helpful. In fact, his collaboration with therapy may be made in a much more indirect way through 'covert' requests. Under the apparent guise of a referral for a patient, these are requests which are actually made on behalf of the team itself.

An oncology unit is a system in perpetual motion and delicate balance, constantly overcharged with emotional tensions and reactions to stress. Distress, failure and frustration, fantasies of death and separation, the high death rate, and the fairly rapid turnover of patients, with perpetual new beginnings, make it necessary to deal with concerns and conflicts as they arise. This is how requests for consultations, which are more often than not indirect requests, reflect the tensions between the vulnerability of the carers, their personal sensitivity, and the daily needs of the patients. All this tension can be dispersed in regular discussions, if possible in a group, where each person can speak about his own feelings and above all about his ambivalence or his feelings of hostility in relation to certain patients. This is a way of sharing and of observing that one is not alone in experiencing the same things. It also allows team relationships to be strengthened by encouraging a feeling of belonging to a structured entity which meets common objectives and concerns. In this setting, the psychiatrist can truly demonstrate his specialist skills of communication and of modelling behaviour.

More simply, it could be said that the anxiety induced by the conditions of stress to which the team is exposed often makes itself felt in terms of interprofessional conflict, and it must be possible to remove the causes of this conflict in terms of the relationship between the patient and the team (Mohl 1980).

– A health-care team always has difficulty in escaping the 'all or nothing' principle. Often, it has the impression either that the patient is too optimistic with regard to the seriousness of his condition, or that he denies it. It is difficult for the team to distinguish between a patient who 'doesn't want to think about that, because it is painful' and a patient who denies reality in a pathological manner. For carers things must be clear, and the ambivalence of patients, or their selective denial, is often difficult to understand.

- Teams sometimes have a stereotyped idea of the role of relatives. Someone will say, for example, 'That woman doesn't behave like a wife', and will adopt a hostile attitude towards her because she is not around her husband enough, or does not kiss him, or because she speaks of his death when nothing of the sort is expected. In this case the team will perhaps have omitted to set the case in context, to imagine what ordeals this woman has already endured, or in what way her husband's pathology may upset her or even revolt her. This might be called a team conflict caused by a transgression of expected roles.
- When they are fighting for survival, teams find it very hard to cope when relatives or patients themselves anticipate death too soon, even if this is sometimes an appropriate reaction. It is customary for carers to deny death so as to continue to believe in what they are doing.
- The situation that is worst tolerated by a team is an aggressive attitude on the part of the patient. We have seen that for some patients, projection, rage or anger were adaptive mechanisms. This sometimes hurts nurses, who feel personally attacked and discredited in their desire to do good. The patient or his relatives may then become scapegoats.
- Physical disablement or the loss of an organic function may be better tolerated by a patient than a state of depression or distress. It is quite the opposite for the team, often consisting of young adults, who will project their own fears with regard to disablement and will imagine that the patient must inevitably be depressed: hence the request for a psychiatrist.
- Discussion groups facilitate the acceptance of patients as they are, mostly 'psychologically normal' people confronted with a very difficult existential situation, in the face of which they react in an individual way. This adaptation to the illness should be seen as far as possible from the biopsychosocial viewpoint.

Defence mechanisms are seen not as barriers to be broken down according to a stereotyped model, but rather as adaptative responses which should be recognized and respected. When he is open to this perspective, the carer within the group can better identify the origin of his own anguish. This also allows him not to lose sight of the fact that the patient's state may be conditioned by exchanges or messages coming from other authorities with whom he will need to co-operate: the family, the ward doctor, but also the laboratory technicians, the radiologists, and the other specialists. At the heart of such a system, the first task of the care-givers is to ensure effective care and a certain quality of life for the patients. This can only be done by bearing in mind the different networks involved. In the course of their journey, patients wander from one sphere to another, or are dependent on several spheres at once. Here is where the psychiatrist can offer interventions which are not only connected with the physiology or the psychodynamic of the individual, but which concern several levels of the institutional organization. This happens, for example, when a patient is hospitalized and the oncologist with whom he has established a significant relationship is only the consultant of the new ward doctor with whom he has to deal. These are difficult situations for patients, which are expressed by symptoms (sleep disorders, anxiety, anorexia) which will be treatable not simply by medication but by analysing the system involved (Barsky and Brown 1982; Eisendrath 1981; Allen 1979).

Chapter 8

Nursing care

A SPECIAL RELATIONSHIP

In hospital out-patient departments, on a daily basis, nurses are in direct contact with their patients and are the best placed to listen to their concerns. These are favourable occasions for developing relationships of trust and also for receiving confidences. In fact, in the eyes of the patient, the doctor occupies a place apart in the therapeutic hierarchy, which will have the corollary that often the patient will avoid bothering the doctor with emotional problems which he feels are of secondary importance or, worse, may risk imperilling the consistency of his care. The patient has a quite special way of protecting his doctor by making all sorts of plausible excuses for him: he is too busy, he is preoccupied with technology, or he is over-tired. On the traditionally feminine side of the team, the nurse (whether male or female) is in a much better position to hear about whatever is going wrong. This is an important aspect of the patient's experience, though it is often hidden because, when he is doubtful, demoralized or distressed, he tends to be afraid that he will not come up to scratch. Poletti makes the following comment:

> The act of nursing is only expressed in the relationship with another person. To care is always to enter into a relationship with a person or a group. To care is to offer to another possibilities of developing his potential and of choosing what is the best action or solution for him, at this moment, in the context in which he finds himself.
>
> (Poletti 1984: 2208)

And it is true that unlike in medical schools, a theory of nursing care is an integral part of the training programme, guaranteeing general coherence. 'The nurse should first of all know her job, and be clear about the nature of her interventions, so as to be able to improve her skills' (Poletti 1984).

But, like doctors, nurses may want to avoid this relationship. They will feel guilty and inadequate because they can do no more, or because they have no way of dealing with what they have noticed. Such feelings will take the form of a certain resentment with regard to the expectations of the patient or his family, or acrimony towards the doctor who is not conducting the case correctly. It is in these circumstances that nurses will become vehement in asking for a drug or a therapeutic procedure that may save the patient; they will take it so much the worse if doctors fail to respond. 'Pseudo-mutual' relationships, over-cordial, may also denote the nurse's own insecurity and her anxiety with regard to cancer and death. Suddenly changing the subject, or rushing out of the room alleging some important errand, are the most usual avoidance activities.

THE TEAM APPROACH

Team case-conferences and exchanges of information facilitate the comparing of actual experiences with regard to the patient, the disease, the prognosis and death. These discussion groups help everybody to understand, to accept his own feelings, and by so doing, even to understand better those of the patient. Comparison is very important, for one discovers that others too can go through phases of frustration, depression, despair or vulnerability. If this exchange does not take place, one discovers that health-care teams imagine that 'good nurses' ought never to have such feelings and that they are condemned to bear everything, beyond the limits of their strength. An interesting phenomenon is that generally the patient's internal problems or conflicts are projected on to the teams as on to a huge screen. The results are interprofessional conflicts, hierarchical confusion, and sometimes contradictory attitudes in the approach to the patient. For example, some young patients suffering from leukaemia, testicular cancer, or Hodgkin's disease may be addressed familiarly and over-indulged by part of the team, even though they may become very dependent and temperamental. On the other hand, another group of nurses may be extremely aggressive and distant towards them. Often the problem will be displaced and seen in terms of skill, fatigue, rotas or the organization of care, which can only make things worse. It is better to realize that nurses, who are often young, are perhaps identifying with the patient, partially fusing with him or on the other hand rejecting him. In doing this they are only unwittingly working through their own emotional problems or issues of autonomy in relation to their parents or family, which happen to be caught up in the disease.

This is also the case when the nurse begins to criticize the therapeutic regime which has been adopted, saying, 'Why are they giving this treatment? He's going to die in any case', or 'Why are people so upset simply because they have cancer?'. There too, without realizing it, nurses represent the hidden face of the case's ambiguity. It is true that when they ask the doctor's help, they are often disappointed. If he has not been able to improve the patient's situation, nurses are often left to themselves, feeling helpless. They do not understand that the skilful and 'all-powerful' doctor can have weaknesses.

At Lausanne, in the multidisciplinary Oncology Centre, we hold regular meetings to relieve the tensions in the team. So as to prevent these discussions becoming group therapy, they are patient-centred, tackling problems first in an intellectual and educational manner. This provides a way of channelling distress and preventing anyone becoming the 'patient' or scapegoat, if he should express too much personal emotion. When trust is established, one can bring out the individual attitudes of the participants more directly. It is not enough to reassure the staff, declaring that their skills are not in question and admitting that the patient is demanding. It is important to encourage them to look at the patient afresh, to suggest practical ways of changing the mode of communication with him, while taking account of the details of his case history and his personal characteristics. In this manner, nurses can make their mode of intervention more flexible and find ways of strengthening their feelings of professional competence. They will finally understand that it is necessary to share their subjective experience with colleagues who are wrestling with the same serious problems.

DEALING WITH STRESS

It must be said that some doctors have ways of protecting themselves and of not becoming involved for long hours with suffering and desperate people. It is not the same for the nursing staff, who stay with patients for a long time and take things to heart. Despite the best intentions, nurses who have too many calls on their time and are overburdened with upsetting information may also end up taking refuge behind a barrage of scrupulously assiduous care. Left to cope with psychological problems on their own, they will perhaps develop a feeling of being all-powerful, which will jeopardize not only their patients but also their private life. They will become rigid, closed to all suggestions, not allowing any change which could be interpreted as a threat to their function. Some works have described, in these cases, functional disorders among nurses as well as the development of emotional problems or even drug abuse (Zumbrunnen 1992).

Finally, as with doctors, the problem arises of nurses knowing how to keep a sufficient distance in order to think and function while being sufficiently near to establish a satisfactory relationship. A common solution is to address the stressful situation in too professional a manner – for example, under the guise of an exclusively technical communication: when one speaks of the 'breast cancer in cubicle 1', the individual becomes a dehumanized object. Quite frequently in our discussion groups, we reduce the tension by resorting to jokes, which is a way of dedramatizing things, within limits. Doctors, in the field of cancer medicine as elsewhere, have gratifying fringe benefits in their hierarchical position, including being able to have exchanges with other colleagues during conferences and trips. I believe that for the members of health-care teams, this recipe is just as valuable; they too must here find satisfaction, positive feedback and rewards. They must be able to follow further training courses, attend conferences or seminars, and obtain simpler rotas and a less rigid work regime.

The basic solution, nevertheless, remains that of exchange, information, respect for one another and the sharing of tasks in an atmosphere of reciprocity. Regular conferences, correct definition of roles and expectations, the working through of unhelpful attitudes and of aggression, which is most often unconsciously induced by patients, remain the best guarantee of maintaining the required therapeutic regime.

A welcome recent development in Britain has been the recruitment of specially trained oncology nurses, the Macmillan nurses, who have an important liaison role and a key part to play in the emotional support of cancer patients.

Chapter 9

Continuity of care

THE GENERAL PRACTITIONER

What has been said above of the doctor applies as much to the general practitioner as to the specialist. The latter cannot, if he carries out the treatment, consider himself only as a scientific expert. The patient will in fact expect much more of him, in proportion to the trust and the responsibility which he invests in him.

For his part, the general practitioner, especially if he has known his patient for a long time, must remain on hand to clarify problems, on request or as the need arises. His role is essential at the start of the illness, for he must find words in which to communicate the diagnosis, but also establish the style of handling the case and the exchange of information with the relatives. He will also know how to offer the space and time necessary to convey the news. This will allow the patient and those close to him to come to terms with what has happened and to prepare themselves mentally for what is to come.

Several interviews are thus necessary (at short intervals) to discuss all the details of the case. The next stage is to find the best way of co-operating with the cancer centre or the specialist concerned (Lee *et al.* 1983).

LIAISON WITH CONSULTANTS

The family doctor should let the specialist know that he has been commissioned to carry out a particular task, to be a partner in therapy, and that he himself wants to continue to be involved in the design of the care plan. Often the patient and his family do not come to consider the specialist as a confidant, and they frequently return to their doctor to seek further explanations and advice about the attitude to adopt when faced with new aspects of the disease or the treatments. For this reason a continued dialogue between GP and consultant is necessary in order to ensure the most effective care (Williams 1983).

This need continues throughout the course of treatment, with the emphasis later shifting towards the quality of life. In fact, the oncology centre sometimes employs the most effective therapeutic plans in a somewhat theoretical manner, and it is only on his return home that the patient will be able to come to terms with the practical implications for everyday life. He will then tend to consult his family doctor urgently, particularly during the days following chemotherapy or radiotherapy. Later, with the worsening of the disease, the patient will be happy to have been able to retain a source of support in the place where he lives, with which he can have direct and rapid contact. This will be particularly necessary in the terminal phase, with its palliative care, when the patient will need to stay at home. But there is also an issue concerning the general policy of care. A further problem is that many side-effects are caused by the conditioning acquired at the hospital at the time of treatment. It is thus desirable that certain therapies be administered in the more pleasant and more intimate atmosphere of the consulting room, where neither the colours, nor the smell, nor the general ambience, nor certain stereotypical remarks recall precisely what triggered the problematic reactions. This also avoids unnecessary fatigue and travel.

CO-ORDINATION OF CARE

This reallocation of tasks requires a co-ordinated policy to avoid fragmentation of care and dispersal of information, which is very likely, given the number of necessary interventions. This is why the concept of a cancer care team is becoming more and more common. The team does not merely collect together the various specialists engaged in the treatment of the disease, but also the representatives of all the psychosocial disciplines. In this way the co-ordination of medical care is assured, but the social and psychological needs of the patient are also not forgotten.

If all the specialists consult each other, at the time of the first assessment of the medical and psychological situation, latent and future problems can possibly be identified and dealt with before crises arise.

The meeting together of several people to tackle a particular problem and to facilitate the sharing of impressions or suggestions does not exclude the absolute necessity for a co-ordinating doctor who centralizes everything and monitors the patient. The team concept is helpful for the biopsychosocial approach and for the dilution of anxiety (the therapist is not alone), but it should not at the same time mean the forgetting of responsibilities and avoidance of the carer–client relationship.

TEAM-BUILDING

The exact composition of the team will vary according to the structure and size of institutions, but also according to geographical considerations, which may or may not favour a dialogue between GPs and specialists. Usually, the team will include representatives of surgery, radiotherapy, medical oncology, psychology, and nursing care.

Nurses, in particular, play an essential part in the team. They see the patient more frequently, at times when he is perhaps more inclined to share his feelings and less preoccupied by purely medical problems. But they are not the only ones, and it would be helpful if more dieticians, physiotherapists, and clergy were to be involved with the physical and spiritual problems of the patient.

Once a team has been set up, its effective functioning is guaranteed by close and frequent communication. The information gained about the physical and emotional state of the patient should be shared among the members. In theory at least, all hierarchical relationships, areas of competence and roles should be frequently redefined, for they are the first structures to disintegrate in the presence of the stress and anguish induced by cancer.

To avoid conflicts, rifts, the categorizing of 'good' and 'bad' patients or 'good' and 'bad' therapists, and also to avoid adopting a too different vocabulary in communicating with the patient, it is necessary to observe a certain number of rules:

- if possible, take account of affinities in team-building;
- avoid having too large a team, and keep other available specialists on call in case of need;
- choose a facilitator not merely according to his hierarchical position, but also for his capacity to make relationships;
- establish ground rules for decision-making;

– make a distinction between decisions that must be taken by everybody (for example, the general policy for treatment) and more technical decisions which must be delegated to the different specialists represented; and
– find a common language.

Chapter 10

Treatments

SURGERY

For a large number of cancers – but also in the minds of many patients – surgery is the first and most effective oncological treatment. The idea of mechanically removing the source of the disease and of cleansing the original location of all evil often seems like a fundamental gesture for patients; they will more readily feel abandoned, or seriously attacked, if an operation is not possible. It might be said that the 'surgical attitude' even corresponds to a way of thinking, since in a certain number of cases we continue to intervene in this way, even when we know that the disease is systemic. In saying that, I do not of course argue against clear indications for oncological surgery.

The desire to be operated upon does not exclude the fact that the patient may feel great anxiety and much distress during the pre-operative period. These reactions are often linked with fears of death, of loss of control in entrusting oneself completely to the care of doctors, and of waking up mutilated, disturbed by narcosis and by pain. Such thoughts frequently give rise to quite violent dreams and nightmares, where the patient visualizes his butchered body, his own death, or that of his relatives. Of course, this scenario may be aggravated by previous experiences of surgery or stories told by relatives.

Pre-operative fears are normal, and even desirable, for they signify that the patient is conscious of what will happen to him and is trying to prepare for it psychologically. Certain studies have shown that patients who do not react, who remain completely impassive and show no sign of depression, are at great risk of presenting post-operative complications at the moment when they become brutally aware of what has happened to them. This is reason enough to encourage preparatory interviews, during which the operative procedure will be carefully explained, with the clearest possible explanation of the indications, the risks incurred, the physical problems expected, and the most long-lasting handicap envisaged. Poor preparation, without speaking of worries, may later give rise to functional disorders, hypochondriacal preoccupations, and even aggression towards the doctor or the hospital team.

Although the anaesthetist and the other members of the team, especially the nurses, may be of great assistance, most of the responsibility falls on the surgeon. In the patient's eyes, he very often remains the only truly significant person at such moments, for only he is sufficiently invested with authority, charisma, and trust to give information to the patient effectively. Such consultations therefore should not be hurried. This avoids any misunderstandings which may arise in the mind of the patient or his family with regard to certain surgical techniques.

Generally, after the operation, the early days are favourable, for the patient has the impression that the danger has receded and that he can detect tangible signs of getting better, whether in observing the healing of the operation wound, the resumption of bowel action, or in taking his first steps in the room and the corridors. It is only later, after the effects of the anaesthetic have worn off, when he has become conscious of his bodily modifications, that the patient will have need of new information to cope with his state. His first concern will be to know if the operation has been successful in removing everything or controlling the disease sufficiently. It may happen, on the other hand, that this is a period when no question is asked, as a necessary latent period of psychological preparation. This can be often seen in women after a mastectomy, who only react at the time when they return home, or who can only accept the idea of having lost their breast several weeks or months after the operation. It is clear that the patient's adaptation to the results of surgery is largely determined by the significance that the organ, or the part of the body affected, had for her or him. It is a matter of the integration and harmonization of the body and spirit, self-esteem and the role of the body in relation to other people. If it is a question of an amputation, the loss of important tissue, an unaccustomed scar or, in the case of ear-nose-and-throat cancers, of an aesthetic change which is difficult to camouflage, the patient's whole social and sexual identity may be called into question.

Many patients will not be able to return to work or keep up their usual performance; they will therefore have the impression of having lost their status or of no longer occupying their place in the family. Other difficulties are well known, notably those arising from dealing with colostomies or urostomies, which are easily disguised but pose problems of evacuation, smell, and noise which disturb social or sexual activity.

For patients who cannot adapt, a problematic gap arises between the body as it now is and the image of it which the patient still has in his mind. This refusal to recognize reality is a form of denial. If it is lifted, this will lead to mourning for the part or the function that has been lost, with the accompanying physical and emotional symptoms. Certain situations have been observed where the amputation of a limb from a very athletic patient, who had a narcissistic investment in his body, gave rise to the appearance of phantom pain, as if to fill an intolerable void in his self-image. This may also arise when a patient is told that there is no further need of medical care.

A similar type of 'filling' empty space may appear in the form of changes in dietary habits (for example, bulimia in a woman who has had a hysterectomy). Such people may also underestimate their true physical and sexual potentialities, experiencing their bodies as much more affected than they really are.

Special attention should be paid to depressive states, to negative emotions and to psychic regressions arising after ablation or amputation of an essential organ or limb. If these feelings cannot be expressed by the patient, they will appear in roundabout ways as pains, losses of function beyond the physical handicap, and difficulties of rehabilitation. There, too, the team can help the patient to adapt, in encouraging continual effort and in possibly involving him in a well-structured programme of rehabilitation, a necessary device for getting him back on his feet and for channelling his distress.

The return home should be carefully organized. Sometimes the mistake is made of thinking that when he is among his own people, the patient will receive the attention and the support he needs. However, it is often the case that leaving hospital is as painful and distressing for him as was his admission. In order to endure hospitalization, mutilating surgery and all the resulting treatments, patients adopt a position of dependence or submission, which is the only way of accepting therapeutic procedures without resistance. It is the search for an infantile stage of security. During this phase, they allow the carers to get on with things, keeping silent about their subjective life or repressing it to some extent, so as to avoid disturbing their relationships with the team and unconsciously avoiding rejection or poor care. To a certain degree, this 'role of the sick person' is useful and normal, but it can change into institutionalization, particularly if, on the surface, the family environment is unstable. Before the patient leaves, therefore, the receiving network outside must be assessed, contact made with the relatives, and the presence of a family doctor ascertained. In certain situations, the organization of a programme of domiciliary care is necessary, with visiting nurses, physiotherapy, or perhaps special meals, especially for patients who live alone.

THE SPECIAL PROBLEM OF BREAST RECONSTRUCTION

To undergo the diagnosis of breast cancer is a traumatic experience, and mastectomy, which is still a common therapy, creates an additional emotional shock. Anguish, a feeling of worthlessness, and depression are the classic reactions, caused as much by the change of body image as by the idea of having cancer.

Women do not all react in the same way, and psychological stress depends on multiple factors, adjustment resulting from the balance found between the development of oneself and one's body image, youthful aspirations and their realization with time, and above all the emotional satisfaction that has been obtained.

It has often been said that the woman must go through the experience of the loss of her breast after the operation, and that this takes time. In fact, after a year or two of disturbance, the patient usually readapts to life and rediscovers a certain pleasure in emotional and social relationships (Asken 1975; Pfefferbaum *et al.* 1977–8).

Certain studies have shown that the least happy women, and those who reject mutilation the most, ask for reconstruction the quickest, as if to neutralize their experience of loss (Maillard *et al.* 1980). It has even been reckoned that the request for reconstruction was a significant indication of non-adaptation. The problem of plastic breast surgery is very controversial. It is difficult to know when to suggest it, even when it presents no technical problem. Apparently, it does not affect survival and is not an obstacle in the way of treating recurrences (Georgiades *et al.* 1985).

For a long time, reconstructions were opposed on the grounds of prudence, for patients may have complaints about the shape, the structure, and odd sensations around the reconstructed breast. There are problems of pain or tugging sensations, but also of claims against surgeons and manufacturers: there have been concerns about long-term product safety. Such problems are not easy to deal with.

Some clinical observations have shown that through their apparently exclusively physical suffering, women are trying to say something to the doctor that goes beyond organic problems (Guex 1986a).

Some women have experienced many difficult times before the appearance of their primary disease (bereavement, separation, lack of fulfilment), or have just been through a tragic experience. Perhaps they were expecting the doctor to effect a more global rehabilitation. Agreement is reached with the doctor about the reconstruction, but the hope that this request represents may go well beyond the technical resources of the surgeon. This is one of the reasons for the delay that should be observed in proposing reconstructions, for finding a new personal balance after such a shock takes time. This move corresponds to the traditional attitude, and the doctor always has a duty to spot those at risk (Staps *et al.* 1985).

At present, fresh enquiries are allowing the debate to widen (Barrett Noone *et al.* 1982). Independently of oncological criteria, which are certainly an important element, it is seen that the delay in reconstruction or the refusal of reconstruction quite often does not really depend on the psychological state of the patient or her sociocultural level, but rather on the information that she will have received from her relatives, other women, or the family doctor. Many of these decisions depend on the doctor and on his capacity for giving objective and detailed information. It is therefore a problem of doctor–patient relationship and of communication. There is hardly ever enough emphasis on this information, which allows women to make informed choices and to express their objections or their anxiety. We certainly know that if they allow themselves to be operated on in full knowledge of the facts, they will afterwards accept much more naturally any inconveniences or imperfections and will have less functional pain. It is significant that women who have been able to prepare themselves for their mastectomy, in discussion with volunteers or with specialist staff, are much less traumatized psychologically. This seems to mean that it is not necessary for them to experience the loss of the breast for a long time (say, one or two years) to be truly aware of the experience and to accept the situation (Dean *et al.* 1983; Stevens *et al.* 1984).

Other results support this statement. Wellisch *et al.* (1985) assessed the psychosocial differences of two groups of women having the same characteristics (age, marital status, socio-economic level). One group received immediate reconstruction, that is to say, in the same operation as the mastectomy. The other group only underwent reconstruction after a year's delay. There was complete correspondence between the two groups as regards aesthetic evaluation of the plastic surgery, which was experienced as satisfactory by 85 per cent, but all the women deplored the loss of an essential sexual attribute, whatever their age. On the other hand, the difference was much greater between the two groups at the level of emotional reactions. The women who had to wait for reconstruction had been through moments of stress, depressive periods, and great perplexity. The others had not been through the same experiences and were less afraid of cancer. Another important element, they did not feel altered in their femininity, their attractiveness, and their possibilities of relationships.

In general, in addition to the comfort that it represents compared with removable prostheses, the maintenance throughout the ordeal of the shape of a breast, even if it is imperfect, diminishes the trauma of the ablation experience and has considerable bearing on the quality of life.

In conclusion, information and support for women faced with this kind of trauma perhaps allows them to be offered the possibility of a reconstruction without unnecessary suffering and yet without their denying what has happened to them (Euster 1979).

RADIOTHERAPY

It is probable that of all the kinds of oncological treatment, radiotherapy is the most surrounded by mystery, fear, and incomprehension. In particular, it is regarded as a treatment which does more harm than good, comparable with urban civilization, car fumes, and above all, with what people say about radioactivity; it seems as if it were a question of treating evil by evil. The thought of undergoing an 'invisible' treatment, immobile under a huge machine, without noise and all alone in a room, frightens the patient and his family in an altogether understandable way. Moreover, undergoing radiotherapy is systematically associated in the mind of the population with the idea of a bad prognosis, even a catastrophic outcome, a state of pitiable decay. But he also has more precise fears, of being burnt, disfigured, or losing essential physiological functions. Everything depends, it seems, on the more or less impressive appearance of the apparatus that is used. Some patients will be convinced that they will be weakened by the treatment, lose their sexual function, or become sterile. For others, the certainty of being contaminated will confirm their feeling of alienation, isolation, and abandonment. An aggravating factor is that most of the time practising doctors are unable to give adequate information on the type of treatments, and many erroneous ideas still circulate. Also, the explanations given by specialists are not always clear and often go beyond people's capacity to understand. In the United States, manuals containing standardized interviews have been published, where the usual concerns of patients are tackled systematically, trying to give appropriate replies which are sufficiently accurate scientifically but not too detailed. When one speaks of the effect of radiation on areas other than the site of the disease, it is helpful if the partner is present, for people tend to associate radiation with sexual and reproductive problems.

It is very important to speak of the modern equipment available, of its capacity to control the dose and to adapt the radiation to each case, with very little risk in the end to healthy tissue. To have a preparatory visit to the radiotherapy department and have preliminary contact with the technical staff can be a good way of preventing future anxieties.

There is no psychosocial approach which is specific to radiotherapy, and the broad guidelines established in the preceding chapters are also applicable here. It is known that, except for certain notable exceptions, radiotherapists have a very particular way of handling relationships with patients and have the tendency, more than others, to take refuge behind their machines. In their defence, it is also true that they often come from disciplines where the relationships are very technical. If they do not feel equipped to play the psychologist, radiotherapists can nonetheless help their patients effectively by attending to their comfort and controlling side-effects such as alimentary problems, nausea, vomiting, and fatigue. Diets rich in calories and proteins can diminish nausea. Balanced nutrition helps one to tolerate the treatment.

To sum up, it may be said that if the patient understands that radiotherapy comes within the framework of a policy of integrated care, and that it has its place under this heading, he will accept it with much more confidence, without automatically imagining that his case is desperate.

CHEMOTHERAPY

The side-effects of chemotherapy cover a wide range, from physical problems to psychological disorders, according to the type of drug used and the particular characteristics of the person who receives it. This is a very specialized field, for the conditions in which the treatment takes place have a great influence on the quality of life and the patient's adaptative mechanisms. It is not enough to tell the patient that chemotherapy is a transitory inconvenience that is likely to prolong his life; he must also be assured that everything will be done to support him during this ordeal. Cytotoxic drugs are often experienced as an intolerable intrusion and an attack on the integrity of the patient, destroying the last vestiges of health in which he might still have confidence.

The cancer patient will often wonder whether the treatment is any use, what are the side-effects, how serious they are, and what other kinds of problems may appear. Carefully conducted interviews can anticipate the patient's questions and lead him to grasp what is expected of him, in return for what benefits for his health. As before, careful explanations should be given about the indications for the treatment, the manner in which it will be administered, how often, and the risks and necessary precautions. The patient should know what is going to happen, without being overwhelmed with ominous prospects. He will be reassured if the carers show their determination to reduce side-effects as far as possible, sometimes by adapting the dosages, by prescribing anti-emetics or tonics, or in teaching certain adjuvant techniques (relaxation, auto-hypnosis, psychological desensitization).

One of the most distressing things for patients, worse than nausea, is the loss of hair. This falling out of whole tufts is sometimes experienced as an intolerable attack on the identity. Some patients testify to having had the impression that their body was disintegrating before their eyes. Few people can withstand the shock of such an ordeal with equanimity, even if they are prepared for it. In every case it is desirable, as much for men as for women, to put them in touch with the wig-maker even before the start of the treatment. We have observed men of a certain age, to whom no one had bothered to mention this problem, who have not left home for six months for fear of frightening the neighbours.

The problems of nutrition, nausea, and vomiting have been touched on earlier. It is clear that they can be relieved up to a point by oral medication and suppositories, but also by means of an appropriate diet. The combination of the stress of cancer and chemotherapy can produce emotional reactions which oscillate from depression or prostration to more euphoric moments. The relatives ought to be told that this has nothing to do with their attitude, but corresponds to the variation of the patient's mood according to his hopes and fears concerning the progression of the disease.

For many young patients, the main fear is that of sterility. Women may have an irregular cycle, and their menstruation may stop altogether. This does not automatically mean that they will be definitely sterile, which is why they should be encouraged to keep up effective contraception. With men, oligospermy or azoospermy is often observed. Generally, this improves with the end of the chemotherapy, but sometimes permanent sterility may result. Sterility is a difficult problem for unmarried people who might want to marry and have children, or for couples who have not yet had them. Carers should think about this and inform men of the possibility of banking sperm for artificial insemination. Explaining all the details of a course of chemotherapy, the side-effects and the ways of alleviating them takes time. The oncologist is the person best placed to speak about all this and to establish a good-quality doctor–patient relationship. This relationship is indispensable to ensure a certain continuity of care and the best possible interpretation of the patient's complaints. In fact, if one has the situation well in hand and if one knows one's patient, it will be easier to assess whether problems are caused by anxiety or by a recurrence. If the therapist changes too often, there is a risk of continually resorting to new investigations, which are distressing, useless, and tiring. In fact, if in doubt, the symptoms that arise are always interpreted in terms of cancer and rarely in terms of mental state.

Whatever the side-effects, it should be remembered that the patient undergoing chemotherapy suffers unusual stress. It is distressing to know that a toxic drug is circulating in one's veins, above all if one does not know exactly what it is doing there. Nausea and vomiting are particularly intense during the first hours or days after treatment. As time passes, problems fade away and the patient feels better. However, this experience leaves its mark not only in the memory but also in the body. This is how, at the time of the next treatment, totally uncontrollable reactions may develop, leading to side-effects, at times even before the drips are in place. I explain elsewhere (see p. 123) how to palliate these acquired behavioural symptoms.

Other side-effects – tiredness, weight loss, and alopecia – come later on, at the time when there is a certain accumulation of drugs in the body. This sets in train the vicious circle described earlier and has the result that the patient never feels really well.

Teams need to have a lot of patience and the ability to listen, to persuade and to maintain, in spite of everything, an atmosphere of confidence. For certain tumours, the visible effects and the subjective improvement which results offer sufficient return for holding on. I am thinking in particular of Hodgkin's disease or other lymphomas where tumoral masses melt like snow in summer, and remarkable progress ensues. It is also the case, for example, with all the pains caused by bony metastases, which, with chemotherapy, disappear almost completely in a short while.

The situation is more problematic for adjuvant treatments, and here much encouragement is needed. In fact, these maintenance treatments, usually administered in situations where the patient feels no symptom of his illness, are difficult to accept, for they offer no peg on which to hang (there is no way of seeing if there is an improvement), and one always wonders about the end-point, as in every chronic situation. The most worrying thing is that the end-point sometimes coincides with death.

To sum up, one could say that the patient undergoing chemotherapy never feels really ill nor completely well, and consequently has a need to keep up close links with the health-care team during the whole course of his treatment.

Chapter 11

Complementary medicine

GENERAL

If orthodox medicine were more effective in curing cancer and in providing supportive care, no doubt patients would rarely seek help from unorthodox practitioners. The available studies indicate that 25 to 45 per cent of patients have recourse to complementary treatments (Guex 1984a). Some turn to unorthodox therapies when orthodox medicine has failed (Bishop 1985) or has nothing further to offer (Thomson 1989), but many use such therapies to complement orthodox treatment in the hope of mitigating side-effects or improving their prognosis or their general health (Arkko *et al.* 1980; Vissing and Petersen 1981; Schraub *et al.* 1982; Guex 1983). Indeed, therapies often classed as 'complementary', such as relaxation and visualization, are available in some orthodox centres as 'adjuvant' treatments (Moorey and Greer 1989).

Definitions

There is a problem of nomenclature, depending on one's point of view and cultural background. In China, Western medicine is combined with traditional medicine (Wenjun 1988), and the doctor advises which treatment is appropriate for each patient; but traditional medicine has its own epistemological framework. Seen as an independent system, therefore, traditional Chinese medicine is alternative to Western medicine, but it is also used to complement it.

In India, Ayurvedic medicine is the only system serving much of the population (Fulder 1988), for whom it is therefore 'mainstream', a system to which Western medicine is 'complementary'. In multicultural societies it is important to respect and understand parallel traditions (Qureshi 1989); the patient's world view is also an element in the clinical picture.

Polarization and antagonism

In the Western world, there has long been controversy between the supporters of mainstream medicine and the founders or the followers of various complementary and alternative therapies (Cooter 1988), who quote case histories of remarkable remissions from cancer (Cameron and Pauling 1979; Gerson 1990) but have found difficulty in convincing scientific colleagues and in gaining sponsorship for clinical trials: 'The resources and facilities to undertake evaluation are not in place' (Monckton 1993). Moreover, most complementary therapies require patient participation over and above mere pill-swallowing and are often used in combination with each other: they are therefore rarely amenable to rigorous testing. But problems of methodology are not insuperable (Lewith and Aldridge 1993; McGourty 1993).

In the United States, the most controversial treatment has long been Laetrile, which clinical trials have so far shown to be ineffective (Broad 1978; Moertel *et al.* 1982). In Europe, similar substances are also in common use (Serocytol, Solomide, Hemotest of Mattei, Cardolezan, to name but a few) (Schraub *et al.* 1982). For many years Iscador (extract of mistletoe) has been widely used in Britain and Europe, originally at the suggestion of Rudolf Steiner, the founder of anthroposophical medicine.

Scheder (1986) carried out a sociological enquiry on the use of alternative medicine in general (not only for cancer problems). Of 954 people from all over French-speaking Switzerland, 90 per cent stated that they had used it, mostly seeking dietary therapy (38 per cent) or a 'strict diet' (24 per cent). In the Netherlands, more and more patients are rejecting orthodox treatments and accepting only alternative regimens, particularly the Moerman diet, which has gathered many adherents (Pruyn *et al.* 1985). Recent British and American studies (Sharma 1992; Eisenberg *et al.* 1993) have also noted substantial numbers of people using non-orthodox medicine.

As far as cancer is concerned, the confusion about research seems to lie in different concepts of the term 'proven therapy', according to the position that people occupy, medical or non-medical. Indeed, what doctors recommend (surgery, radiotherapy, chemotherapy) may be seen by patients as disastrous, by reason of the unpredictable and sometimes devastating side-effects which they cause, and as offering no guarantee of long-term success.

The debate is for the moment unresolved, for the opposing arguments are not on the same logical plane. On one side, the faculties of medicine argue in terms of experimental work and statistics; on the other, alternative practitioners preach their convictions with a crusading spirit. But to quote Dr Richard Tonkin:

> The imperative for research is now recognised by the main body of complementary therapists and a substantial proportion of the orthodox establishment has at long last become aware of the hidden potential of some of the less scientifically explicable ways of fostering health and dealing with illness.
>
> (Tonkin in Monckton 1993: 5)

PARTNERSHIP WITH THE PATIENT

At all events, doctors must not persist in affirming the superiority of their methods over non-conventional methods, or they will seriously undermine their own credibility. It is simpler to say that some of the remedies of orthodox medicine belong to a certain established order of things and that they have already demonstrated their efficacy for many patients in Europe and the United States.

This indeed presents a significant problem of communication, which should be kept as open as possible, by reason of the defensive actions of consumers who often, rightly, call authority figures into question in order to preserve as far as possible the interests of their members (Holland 1981). Medicine cannot escape this.

From this point of view, the traditional doctor–patient relationship, of power and knowledge on one hand and of dependence and submission on the other, needs to be modified. Indeed, it is not a question of unsettling the patient by allowing him to be the sole judge of the proposed therapies, but on the contrary of empowering and supporting him by giving him the role of partner in the management of his disease. Cancer patients, especially, have need of this, for they are anxious, easily alarmed, and constantly fear loss of control (Spielberger 1975). They thus wish for and have need of information and certainties that often cannot be offered to them. To be able to tackle this kind of problem openly is a sign of an adult relationship, and can only reinforce the atmosphere of trust. And this, I would even say, will allow one to avoid the confrontational situations which are precisely those that encourage the recourse to alternative medicine (Brohn 1986).

Why do patients seek unorthodox treatments?

Epstein (1976) has shown that the most fragile patients, that is, those with the lowest self-esteem, sometimes assimilate information given by the doctor in an incomplete and muddled way. As a result they often appear dissatisfied with their management and are thus more prone to seek answers in non-conventional methods. It is the same for those who respond to emotional shock with anger and conflict.

Pruyn *et al.* (1985) analysed the profile of patients who adopted the Moerman diet. They noted that most of them made their choice because they reckoned they had received insufficient and ambiguous information, which frustrated their need for certainty. At the level of personality, they were very sensitive to threats of every kind, had low self-esteem, and had poor control of their aggressive impulses.

One might deduce that people react badly when they are faced with argumentative patients, and tend to neglect them. On the other hand, impulsive patients have a limited tolerance of frustration and easily take hasty decisions, going elsewhere rather than waiting for hypothetical future improvements.

But it is perhaps helpful to go further and try to grasp what patients are looking for 'symbolically' in this 'otherness', contrasted with official institutions. A certain openness of spirit might perhaps allow doctors to be more tolerant and to accept a more global way of seeing the body and medicine itself, which would send us back to ourselves and to our relationship with the disease.

Cancer generates a huge movement of self-reliance, of concentration of energy and strength in the face of multiple agonizing commitments. It is not by chance that one speaks of fundamental fears, as if one were re-experiencing something of the original fear of being born. Indeed, cancer involves not only an individual illness, but also something about the order of society, the contrasts which we experience between urban civilization and the countryside, between the concrete jungle and nature: something which produces a nostalgia for origins where all was mythically clean and tidy and which would be the last resort for a chance of healing. In the same way as primitive societies with their fear of natural phenomena (storms, forests, sky) have need of magical help, our fear is inexpressible in the face of something alien which, coming from elsewhere, has penetrated the healthy body to harm it – that is, cancer.

The patient is perhaps intellectually equipped to understand the logical propositions of the doctors, but he does not there find his answer at gut-level. Intuitively, and perhaps without altogether realizing it, he will search desperately for salvation so as to escape tragedy. Resorting to complementary medicine is perhaps an attempt to revert to traditional remedies, those of the origins and roots of humanity. Western representatives of complementary medicine, at least for the most part, no longer belong to this kind of tradition, but their offer of global care is perhaps a relic of it.

THE BACKGROUND OF TRADITIONAL MEDICINE

Natural or traditional medicine, for each nation, comes within the scope of a much wider panorama than the limits of the body. The administration of medicines is inseparable from the traditional theory which interprets the phenomena of the world and the functions of man and those of his environment as the result of interaction between opposites. These are two or more complementary principles of one and the same reality. To use a fashionable term, we are talking about holistic medicine.

The notation can be binary – hot/cold, dry/wet, good/bad, yin/yang among the Chinese. In certain countries, as certainly in China (Wenjun 1988), traditional medicine is still widely used and apparently effective. In Puerto Rico, as in China, traditional medicine is combined with Western medicine, retaining a binary hot/cold system of notation. Disease, of which the aetiology is often seen as supernatural, is experienced as an imbalance of the fundamental elements, which will have to be treated by opposites: this treatment is often effected by a rapid transition from hot to cold or vice versa. For example, the treatment of appendicitis, a cold malady, should be done by heat. Present-day drugs are also integrated; penicillin is 'hot' by reason of the warm effects which it occasions, such as diarrhoea; it will be neutralized by mixing it with a 'cold' substance, fruit juice for example (Harwood 1971; Schnorrenberger 1979).

In China, organic and functional elements, subjective and objective, matter and energy, the psychic and the physical, are intimately bound up in the whole medical terminology. In the theory of the meridians of acupuncture, the interior of the body is joined with the exterior and with the cosmos (Boudon 1979).

Here we come near to the medicine of the ancients like Hippocrates and Empedocles, in which the four humours (blood, phlegm, yellow bile and black bile) are mixed in given quantities to ensure health (Lichtenthaeler 1978). Certain traditions have been maintained up to our own time, not only in the composition of basic medicines on natural principles, but also in practice and vocabulary: the head or the stomach is 'burning', or we talk about 'catching cold'. The return to balance is constantly evoked (Schraub et al. 1982).

The goal is then to rediscover inner harmony, the balance corresponding to the context in which one evolves. In order to re-establish this balance, one has recourse to treatments, vegetables, herbs, plants and diets, not so much in a search for remedies that are efficacious or proven but rather so as to return symbolically to tradition, to one's roots, to harmony (Lévi-Strauss 1966); and so to struggle against the passing of time, and even death itself.

In this way one can seek for health in the return to origins, and the 'healer' is invested with a wider role. The repository of knowledge and popular beliefs, he is concerned less with diseases than with people; one may perhaps seek healing from him, but also a possibility of communicating, confiding, and reuniting with one's ancestors.

To gain a privileged relationship with the healer, in a natural and individualized setting, is perhaps to grasp the realization of being fully alive, that the body is the arena of things other than forecasts of death discovered by a doctor. The healer–patient contract, freely chosen by the latter, allows him to enter a field where he may feel alive and active, take charge of his body and his fate, and experience the relief of distress. This step allows the patient to feel no longer alone and to find his place again in a wider whole where the prospect of death perhaps becomes more tolerable (Eliade 1978).

TOWARDS INTEGRATION

To conclude, complementary therapies must not be rejected by endless scientific arguments. In any case, the history of medicine shows that the heterodoxy of one generation often becomes the orthodoxy of the next: healthy scepticism must not rule out open-mindedness. On the contrary, we must try to understand better what is happening, to integrate the subjective space which complementary medicine may occupy, to improve the interpersonal dimension of our consultations, and to listen to patients. It is important to respect the patient's autonomy and to encourage his desire to explore therapies that may help him to feel better (Cosh and Sikora 1989), even if they have no impact on his prognosis. If we condemn complementary therapies, the patient will simply have recourse to them without telling us (Eisenberg *et al.* 1993).

SOME COMPLEMENTARY THERAPIES

Finally, it is worth listing some complementary therapies not mentioned elsewhere in this book that may have a contribution to make to the management of cancer, or to improving patients' quality of life. The list is by no means exhaustive but concentrates on those most commonly used. Manipulative techniques such as chiropractic and osteopathy are not included, as they would not usually be recommended for cancer patients (except for pre-existing conditions) in cases where bone pain might indicate the presence of skeletal tumours.

Acupuncture

Acupuncture was introduced to the West by the French and has been widely practised in French hospitals. In Britain, a substantial minority of conventionally trained doctors have also trained in acupuncture, and there are similar numbers of lay acupuncturists (Saks 1992). The whole person is treated rather than the disease, and no acupuncturist would attempt to insert needles into tumours, but the role of acupuncture as an anti-emetic and for pain relief has been well researched (Dundee 1988; Richardson and Vincent 1986), and it is offered in some hospices. It may also be of benefit in treating post-operative lesions.

Alexander technique

F.M. Alexander, an Australian actor, began to use body work with his colleagues in 1894, and the system (Alexander 1932) is now widely taught in drama and music colleges. Its therapeutic benefits include relief from stress-related disorders, anxiety and depression (Barlow 1973), and rehabilitation after surgery, particularly that affecting the voice (Jones 1976; Stevens 1987). Alexander went to London at the turn of the century and taught in both England and the

United States until 1955. Moshe Feldenkrais combined some aspects of the Alexander technique with oriental body training, and his system is popular in the United States (Feldenkrais 1972). For a detailed description of the 'eutony' of Gerda Alexander which is used in Switzerland, see Chapter 12 under 'Body work'. (G. Alexander is a Danish practitioner and no relation to F.M. Alexander.)

Anthroposophical medicine

Anthroposophical medicine is based on the work of Rudolf Steiner (1861–1925), whose description of man included the spiritual as well as the physical. Though not a medical practitioner he worked closely with doctors (Twentyman 1989). Anthroposophical medicine is part of a wider movement responsible for pioneering work in other fields such as education and the arts, and is particularly well developed in Switzerland, Germany and the Netherlands. It is not alternative to but an extension of scientific medicine (Fulder 1988). Therapies include diets, massage, hydrotherapy, eurythmy, and artistic therapies. Most medicines are from natural sources; the anti-cancer activity of Iscador (from mistletoe) has been the subject of a good deal of controversy (Khwaja *et al.* 1986), but it is available in Britain on National Health Service (NHS) prescription. Anthroposophical physicians, who must be fully qualified doctors, are very much involved in palliative care.

Aromatherapy

This is a form of massage which uses essential oils of flowers and plants, whose perfume may also be of therapeutic benefit on the emotional level, producing a feeling of well-being. Massage eases tension and anxiety (McKechnie *et al.* 1983), increases circulation, stimulates the lymphatic system, and helps to break down scar tissue. It is of particular value in post-operative rehabilitation (for instance in preventing lymphoedema or treating fibrosis), and is sometimes offered in cancer hospitals and hospices in addition to physiotherapy.

Art therapies

Painting, modelling, sculpture and music can be useful adjuncts to psychotherapy, offering powerful non-verbal means of self-expression, rediscovery of one's creative capacities, and communication with others (Liebmann 1986). Art therapy is sometimes offered in cancer hospitals (Connell 1992). Group work, especially in music, has great potential for releasing emotion and does not require prior musical literacy or technique (Alvin 1975; Mandel 1991; Storr 1992).

Ayurveda

Ayurveda, or 'the science of life', with its offshoots Unani Tibb (in Pakistan) and Siddha, is the ancient art of Indian medicine, dating from the fifth century BC, and is practised in Western countries where there are Asian communities. An example of the influence of Ayurveda on Western medicine is provided by the work of the endocrinologist Deepak Chopra, founding president of the American Association of Ayurvedic Medicine, who uses the methods of Ayurveda (dietary change, herbal remedies, yoga exercises, and meditation) alongside conventional chemotherapy (Chopra 1989).

Healing

Healing through prayer or the laying-on of hands has played a part in all religious traditions since primitive times (Pullar 1988), and most modern practitioners claim only to be the channel for the healing power of God: healers who give out their own energy are often left feeling exhausted (Fulder 1988). Anecdotally, healing has benefited cancer patients, who often seek help only when the disease is terminal (Magarey 1981). Where cure is impossible, healing may nevertheless relieve pain and distress (Cadwell 1986) and does not necessarily require faith on the part of the patient, though receptivity is helpful. The aim is to restore the person to wholeness of body, mind and spirit (MacNutt 1974, 1977).

Herbalism

All over the world, modern anti-cancer drugs exist side by side with herbal medicines, from which they may be derived (vincristine, for example, from periwinkle), and in village society health care is largely herbal (Bannerman et al. 1983). Some Western doctors are trained in medical herbalism, and lay herbalists may work alongside doctors. Cancer patients should be encouraged to consult a trained practitioner before taking herbal remedies, which are by no means always innocuous and which should be individually prescribed except for minor ailments.

Homoeopathy

Homoeopathy, originated by Samuel Hahnemann (1842), offers a genuinely alternative medical system, which in its use of minute doses of remedies in high dilutions runs counter to orthodox drug therapy. However, it is often used by orthodox doctors, especially in France, where homoeopathic prescriptions qualify for a state subsidy. It has enjoyed high status in Britain since the early nineteenth century, is practised by many doctors, and may be used as an adjunct to mainstream cancer treatments (Blackie 1986; Clover 1992; Kleijnen *et al.* 1991). Dr Edward Bach developed a variant of Hahnemann's homoeopathy in the form of flower remedies, which are designed to treat the psychological roots of disease (Weeks 1940). Referral to homoeopathic hospitals in Britain may be made by general practitioners working within the NHS, under which treatment is free.

Meditation

The union of the soul with the universal spirit is the goal of spiritual exercises in religious traditions the world over, and meditative techniques can be learnt from a teacher or from books or tapes. Body awareness, such as is experienced in yoga, t'ai chi, or through simple relaxation exercises, may be a precondition for meditation or may provide a meditative experience in itself. The benefits of meditation have been observed (Benson *et al.* 1974; Benson 1975; Meares 1980, 1981; Magarey 1983), and to set aside a regular time for meditation may be a way for patients to validate their own needs and to find peace.

Nutritional therapies

Since it is possible that diet may play some part, among other factors, in the aetiology of cancer (Doll and Peto 1981; Palmer and Bakshi 1983), making dietary changes enables the patient to feel he is doing something to help himself, over which he has personal control. The recommendations of various dietary schools of thought (Moerman, Gerson, Kelley, and others) are similar: usually a vegetarian (sometimes vegan), wholefood, high-fibre regime, with low fat, salt, and sugar. The role of nutritional therapy as curative remains controversial, but as an aid to a generally healthy life-style, to help prevent recurrences, to improve prognosis (Holm *et al.* 1993), and to reduce side-effects of orthodox treatment (Lechner and Kronberger 1990), it may be of benefit. Vitamin and mineral supplements (e.g. vitamin C, beta-carotene, zinc, and selenium) are often recommended in conjunction with dietary regimes (vitamin B12 is indicated when following a fully vegan diet), and in Britain these are available on NHS prescription.

Reflexology

Reflexology, or reflex zone therapy, is a form of foot massage of pressure points in which effects can be brought about in other zones or parts of the body. It has been used for thousands of years in China and Egypt, and was also known to American Indians and some African tribes. Stiffness, tension and stress may be helped by reflexology, which should be given by a trained practitioner (Fulder 1988; Hall 1991). Since only the feet (and sometimes the hands) are massaged, it can be administered in hospital contexts without upsetting ward routines; many nurses have acquired the necessary training, especially in Switzerland, where it is much appreciated.

Yoga and t'ai chi

Yoga, in the ancient Indian tradition, is not a therapeutic science, but 'a science for liberating the soul by bringing the consciousness, the mind and the body to a state of integration' (Iyengar 1988). Health, happiness and healing, however, are seen as by-products. The breathing techniques and exercises of yoga may well be of benefit in post-operative rehabilitation, though certain postures may be unsuitable for particular patients, who should tell their teachers about any disability. Yoga is not competitive, and each participant works at his own pace. T'ai chi is a comparable system of exercises, in the Chinese tradition, which is rather less strenuous and more akin to dance.

To sum up, complementary therapies, whether provided as part of standard hospital treatment, funded by general practitioners, or sought by patients on their own initiative, are forming an increasingly important and indeed popular element in multidisciplinary cancer care. Palliative treatment needs to begin from the time of diagnosis, and should not be confined simply to the terminal phase. By welcoming and supporting this development we are more likely to ensure that the highest standards are maintained among complementary practitioners.

Chapter 12

The psychosocial approach

GENERAL

When his health is seriously under attack, the human being has need of affection, approval and security. He must feel that he is a member of a group where exchanges are fruitful and where there is trust. People who maintain significant social and emotional relationships seem to be better able to bear the physical and emotional shock of disease. They are able to share their feelings and their anxieties, and correspondingly appreciate the help that is offered. The social context provides the patient with a protective and stable environment, in the shelter of which he progressively adapts his way of being and his relationships with the outside world. Affective bonds guarantee his self-respect (his healthy narcissism) in the face of aggressive treatments, physical mutilation, modification of social status, and other setbacks brought about by the cancer (particularly the passage from the state of health to that of sickness).

It is generally agreed that the capacity of people to maintain their psychological equilibrium depends not only on their personal resources but, in an equally important way, on the context in which they develop (Mechanic 1974). Weisman and Sobel (1979) incline to this view, in stating that 50 per cent of the psychological problems reactive to cancer may be improved by non-medical means. Patients indeed seem to live longer if they can keep active and retain enriching affective relationships, compared with those who are without resources and wish to die (the 'giving-up syndrome').

At the level of intervention, it is easier to organize psychosocial management, to improve communication networks and the style of adaptation to the disease, than to change stress factors and personality traits (Gottlieb 1981).

It has not so far been possible to determine clearly who benefits the most from support, nor on which aspect the emphasis should ideally be placed to help cancer patients: should the help be individual or familial, financial or medical? It seems certain, at any rate, that the quality of interpersonal relationships (or even their mere existence) protects people against the effects of stress, prevents physical and mental problems, and improves symptomatology. The human being feels better from the moment when he recognizes himself and is recognized in his perceptions and his affects, if he can continue to tell his story (even if its end is in sight) and if he has the feeling of belonging to a structured group (family, friends, health-care team).

In every case, the doctor and the relatives must avoid hiding behind a stereotyped attitude which is the same for everybody. Every individual element should be taken into account. By carefully considering the challenges that must confront the patient faced with the various stages of treatment, it is possible to plan the most effective strategies. According to the degree of physical disease, age, sex, work and family responsibilities, but also sociocultural level, the patient will expect more or less help. Interventions should allow difficulties to be dealt with in reality but also at the level of subjective experience, above all if the feelings are negative (aggression, anger, revulsion, guilt) (Wortman and Dunkel-Schetter 1979; Silver and Wortman 1980).

The role of families, partners and friends is fundamental, but most studies show that the most important person is still always the doctor. Another important factor is the possibility of sharing with those who are going through the same experience, for example in groups of patients and volunteers (say, breast-care groups or colostomy groups).

Before acting, the doctor should always identify the resources available among the extended family and friends, locating the significant persons. Indeed, he is sometimes over-solicited by the partner, but it may be by a friend or a distant relation who seems to want to take over and who seriously complicates consultations. The doctor's immediate instinct is to keep them at a distance so as not to enter into rivalry with them and so as to give more space to the patient and to his own wishes. But it has to be said straight away that it is just those people who are indispensable to the patient and who will perhaps be the essential source of support around which the doctor can build his intervention.

The analysis of the social context of the patient should take account of the following elements:

- the marital situation;
- participation in sociocultural activities;
- the general organization of life; and
- the way in which the patient refers to others, which is an indirect indication of psychological behaviour (projection, subtle denigration, idealization, isolation, conflict).

People who have few social relationships have a mortality risk that is twice the average (House *et al.* 1982).

Several questions arise. Is it the social support as such which is useful, or simply the effect of relationships which it offers? And if it is the social support, is it its density, its availability or its stability which is the determining factor? A good way of establishing the answers to these questions is to find out what impact the cancer has had: how have things been upset, who has been mobilized or, on the other hand, who has fled, and what changes have come about within the relationships with family and friends?

The reverse of the coin in the context of 'being useful' is that, most of the time, relatives do not know what they ought to do to help the patient. Instead of letting him speak, listening to him, and putting themselves to some extent in his shoes, there are many who cling to clichés in order to contain their own anguish and their fear of emptiness. Relatives or partners are often ambivalent, reassuring on the surface but giving out all sorts of indirect messages that are negative and contradictory. If it is postulated that cancer patients establish unequal and non-reciprocal relationships, it is easy to see that this leads to lack of comprehension. Falsely optimistic phrases proliferate: 'we must all pull together', 'I'm sure everything's going to be all right', 'it's nothing serious', and so on. These phrases take no account of the true relational and affective experience which the relatives and the patient have accumulated. This has the result that feelings of isolation and distress are intensified (Peters-Golden 1982).

Often, the family does not allow the patient to talk about his illness and prevents him from tackling difficulties. On the contrary, they take over everything, undermining the patient's self-confidence and giving him the idea that he is an outcast or plague-stricken. Attitudes of encouragement, established according to a ready-made notion that people have of the situation, are thus often badly received. Patients have a horror of good intentions (Silver and Wortman 1980), which is why it is often simpler to let them go at their own speed and wait for their often painful interrogations and entreaties. False hopes are experienced as a momentary support, but also get in the way of affective movement. It has been observed that the request for help formulated by a patient is a good sign of adaptability. Some people are capable of mobilizing their relatives in times of crisis and of letting their doctor in where they want to. These are the 'good' cases, who know how to defend their interests and who generally benefit the most from the available resources (counselling, support, training) by using them. On the other hand, others, and notably those who correspond to some extent with the psychological profile of the cancer-prone person defined in Table 1.1 in Chapter 1, in spite of themselves, put themselves in the position of irritating their carers, of making them hostile or feel inadequate or insufficient (Silberfarb *et al.* 1980b). These are the people who are at high risk from the point of view of both physical and psychological prognoses.

Would it be possible to find out why those who have the most need are the least in a position to receive help? Will lack of support actually contribute to a poor disease outcome, independently of other stress factors? Or is it that this acts in synergy with the other stressors to produce a poor outcome?

We have the impression that support not only contributes to well-being but may also protect at a more physiological level against the harmful effects of stress. For the moment we do not know what the triggering mechanism may be. Perhaps comfort modifies the perception of stress factors and reinforces the strategies of adaptation.

Table 12.1 Identification of the elements of psychosocial evaluation

1	Observe how the patient expresses his feelings.
2	Try to get an idea of his system of values or his convictions (for example, has he an idea about cancer or about ways of treating it?).
3	Encourage the patient to express his feelings or his convictions freely.
4	Adapt and offer new and diverse information.
5	Evaluate the socio-affective and work-related network of the patient (for example, in which system of loyalties and reciprocity is he involved, which is significant for him?).
6	Encourage problem-solving and receiving practical help.

VARIOUS INTERVENTIONS

Support for the cancer patient has long been synonymous with preparation for death. That remains an important chapter, of course, but at present there is no longer a question of being limited only to situations of crisis and urgency but, while taking account of the progress of the treatment, of helping people to live while adapting to a chronic disease. Everything must therefore be done to avoid patients feeling threatened exclusively by a death sentence.

It has been shown, in particular, that the most difficult time is not the terminal phase but that of the first recurrence after a period of remission (Silberfarb *et al.* 1983). Patients often ask themselves simple questions which have little to do with death. They wonder how they will be able to cope with daily life: 'How will I be able to do the housework?', 'The continual hospital appointments are upsetting my work and my emotional life – what can I do?' and so on. To adapt is a struggle to find an acceptable compromise between contradictory constraints, rather than the attempt to triumph over adversity. A number of patients do not need the help of a professional to do this and manage very well with their own resources (Weisman cited by Goldberg and Cullen 1985). Others request our interventions, which we must be able to adapt judiciously.

'Support' is a fairly vague concept. The most usual types of support are intellectual (cognitive) and social. As new matters arise, the how and the why of clinical and therapeutic procedures should be clearly and systematically explained (Peteet 1982).

Socially, support is respect for a certain quality of life of the patient, while putting at his disposal practical means (transport, social security, financial support, etc.).

Psychologically, there are several ways of offering support:

– *Treatment of psychiatric disorders.* It is important to know how to diagnose and detect the main cognitive disorders, depression and anxiety, in order to treat them, possibly by having recourse to psychopharmacology (Gordon *et al.* 1980). When they have difficulties with memory or concentration, patients do not easily accept that they have problems, which often only appear belatedly, in the form of behavioural disorders (Silberfarb *et al.* 1983).
– *Psychotherapeutic support.* This is expressed in terms of a relationship which gives the patient a feeling of comfort and of respite, a

guarantee of his worth, and the certainty of being respected and valued. Such a relationship allows the patient at least to have a grip on life, even if not on his disease. It also reinforces his feeling of being alive, in reviewing his experience and his emotional bonds.

Psychotherapeutic support can take several forms:
- selective intervention (dealing with a crisis situation);
- individual psychotherapy; and
- group therapy.
- *Cognitive-behavioural methods.* These are centred on a precise task, but they can also be considered from a psychotherapeutic perspective, for they are effective as a confidence-building exercise before undertaking further therapy: certain patients have a need to see the practical usefulness of the therapist's work (Moorey and Greer 1989).
- *Physical techniques.* These encourage relaxation, work on the side-effects of treatments, and allow one to regain a certain control over one's body.

INDIVIDUAL PSYCHOTHERAPY

The management of a cancer patient on the psychological plane sometimes seems a thankless and difficult undertaking. As I have indicated earlier, the questions are: what should one support, and from which perspective; how can one be helpful; and, finally, what should one hang on to, if everything in the sphere of 'action' or 'the possible' is in the hands of the treating doctors (oncologists, surgeons, radiotherapists) (Forester *et al.* 1985).

Sympathy or understanding are not enough in themselves, for they have the tendency to reinforce the patient's feelings of isolation and depression, and he is driven back to the disease itself by this kind of attitude. On the other hand, to make a complete abstraction of cancer, as is sometimes advised, is a trifle unrealistic, for if someone asks for a consultation it is no doubt because he is a prey to real worries about the disease, its progression, and his prognosis. The psychotherapeutic approach perhaps lies between these two, where the therapist, while keeping a certain distance and controlling his own distress and negative attitudes, offers an intermediate space between the family and the health-care team, where the patient can talk and reflect. Here is sought a different kind of rhythm and time from that of medicine. The patient will perhaps be able to find here a wider, less 'stuck' perspective, and calmly decide how best to manage the whole situation.

In contrast to what he does in classical psychotherapy, the therapist should know how to be fairly active, and not be afraid of going beyond the allotted time or of being available when the patient feels he has need of him. He should even sometimes intervene with his colleagues, to inform them and encourage them to take better account of the patient's needs.

It has happened with me, for example, that I have asked for chemotherapy to be postponed because it was to take place at a bad time; called for a fresh interview to clarify matters between the oncologist and the patient; or proposed to the treating physician a complementary examination (a mammogram or a scan) because a patient was extremely anxious about a new symptom and no amount of reassurance could pacify her. (This examination was not perhaps envisaged at that moment in the protocol, but did not actually prove to be a waste of time or money.)

The psychiatrist may thus be the guarantor of a certain quality of care. He will make himself the patient's advocate, and will regularly discuss and review the problems which interfere with his personal functioning and that of his family relationships, his work, and everything that is relevant to his coping with the disease.

Such a partnership allows the patient to retain as much control as possible over what happens to him, in an atmosphere of respect for his feelings. In this way he preserves his individuality and his equilibrium in the face of treatment, relieving the stress associated with the cancer. He can better accept the real threat, helped by a therapist whose presence and commitment to his interests reassure him. To introduce again the terms used elsewhere, we have here an active struggle against hopelessness/helplessness (Tarnower 1984).

This support is sometimes useful in the short term to deal with a crisis situation, or in the long term to give comprehensive support to a patient who is particularly needy, as the two following examples illustrate.

Case study no. 1

Mme V. was 45 years old. Of country stock, she had devoted herself mainly to her task as daughter, then as wife and mother of farmers (she had two adult sons). Having a sense of duty and of self-sacrifice, she was the pivot of all the domestic and family activity of the three generations who lived together. It was discovered that she was suffering from widely metastatic breast cancer, for which she had only sought advice belatedly, after she had observed a swelling for a very long time. She was extremely annoyed that the doctors had taken three weeks to communicate the diagnosis to her. She thought that they had not done their duty, had made errors of interpretation, and that this had harmed her. She submitted reluctantly to chemotherapy, arguing about every move and every decision. She never stopped making comparisons with relatives who had been through severe difficulties, she said, because of their treatments, and all for nothing, since in any case they had died of their cancer.

At the moment when the doctors decided, after two years of chemotherapy, that the disease was in remission and that no further treatment was necessary for the time being, Mme V. requested urgent hospitalization for violent facial pains. All the results of the investigations that were carried out (scan, ENT and neurological examinations) were normal, but the pain persisted and did not respond to any treatment. The patient refused all psychiatric intervention, pointing out that she was not mad and that her mother had been treated as a depressive for a long time before a tumour was discovered, in the same way. Mme V. was then referred to a multidisciplinary pain clinic which had a psychiatrist in the team. The verdict was that she was very depressed and extremely distressed, convinced that her life was at an end. The facial pain perhaps meant that she was coming to the end of her tether, but also that she had a grudge against us.

In more lengthy discussions with her, it was discovered that at one point an oncologist had said to her, on the subject of her bony metastases, that increase of pain would indicate the possibility of increasing the dose of antimitotics, and that this was a good yardstick by which to evaluate the effectiveness of the treatment. After appropriate administration of anxiolytics and antidepressants, it was easy to review calmly with her the problem of her desire to continue the oncological treatment, and to analyse her feeling of being suddenly abandoned. It was then possible to explain under more favourable conditions the reasons for the interruption of the treatment, which enormously relieved her. The decision was even made to resume maintenance chemotherapy, a solution which was considered feasible but had been abandoned, in the belief that this would please her. With a new confidence, she then began to talk about the real problem, which was the marriage of her elder son, and about the conflict that had arisen at the farm with the grandfather, who had not yet given up his place to his own son when the grandson was demanding to take over everything. It was understandable that the exacerbation of her complaints, coming at a turning-point, was also the symptom of her husband's distress. In requesting urgent hospitalization, she was not only reopening the question of oncological treatment but was also offering a breathing-space to all the family as it faced the problem of inheritance.

In this type of intervention, the therapist facilitates the clarification of the situation, the understanding of the symptom reframed in its context, and the search for practical solutions, that is, a precise task. If the patient is agreeable, he can possibly go on to speak of deeper preoccupations or resentments. For this patient, it was possible, in the course of the subsequent sessions, to tackle her feelings of aggression and jealousy towards the relatives who would survive her and over whom she could no longer exercise control.

Case study no. 2

Mr S. was 35 years old. He had been followed for five years by the psychiatrist attached to the oncology department, where he had been treated for a recurrent widespread Hodgkin's lymphoma. His story was not commonplace: being disabled, during his youth he underwent eighteen operations to correct the results of poliomyelitis (occurring at the age of 2). At the start of the treatment, he had already spent two-thirds of his life in hospital. A mixed tumour with multicentric sites was discovered two years after a car accident in which he had caused the death of his passengers. Christened 'the killer' in his locality, he had been forced to uproot himself and migrate to another part of the country, where he had found an administrative job. Though his excellent professional capabilities (resulting from a tremendous effort of social integration) had always been recognized, he found himself perpetually at loggerheads with his boss. In fact, he was considered sometimes as a 'tolerated' invalid, at other times as someone who could be abused by being overloaded, which corresponded exactly to his difficulty in not being really able to accept himself as disabled.

The first meeting with the psychiatrist took place at the time of an episode of exogenous psychosis linked with the first chemotherapy treatment. The patient then refused to continue the treatment, which put him in great danger of general metastasis. The atmosphere with the health-care team was, of course, quite contentious. The intervention first of all allowed the doctor–patient relationship to be clarified and the needs, demands and fears of the patient to be better understood. It was also possible to grasp much better how he felt about his self-image.

The psychotic episode, caused by the toxic effect of the drug used, had been preceded by an event minor in itself but very traumatizing for the patient. In fact, part of the first dose of antimitotics had been injected at the side of the vein and had caused a burn. Generally, people are disagreeably surprised by this kind of thing, but do not have any particular psychological reactions. It was quite otherwise for this patient, whose only really sound limb had been damaged. This was a direct and intolerable attack on his already very disturbed body image. But this also reactivated all the frustrations and unexpressed rage about the malevolence of fate and, of course, of doctors, major figures of his existence on whom he had almost always depended.

It was only possible to continue the treatment by scrupulously ensuring that the patient was always put in the most favourable and reassuring conditions and did not have to suffer the least uncertainty. This management was crucial for his therapeutic opening-up, for which he would have been extremely unready beforehand. From then on, he kept in contact with the psychiatrist, uncovering by stages the story of his handicap, what he had endured and overcome, his permanent flirtation with death and his struggle to escape it. The most dramatic moment was the recalling of the episode of the death of his friends and of the guilt which was eating away at him. He himself made a direct link with the appearance of his cancer. In his eyes it was the price he paid for surviving, in suffering not only the disease, but also the ghetto at his place of work, where he felt trapped.

Over the course of years, in spite of a fairly serious recurrence, involving fresh surgical intervention, it was possible for him to climb steadily back up the slope, while maintaining a very strong bond with the therapist as a point of orientation. Finally, by leaving his place of work and moving to another town, in complete remission, he began to flourish in social and creative activity.

Interventions can be much shorter when, confronted with a 'blocked' situation, we come to appreciate the way in which the patient imagines things, and we modify our attitude accordingly.

Case study no. 3

A patient of 52 years, suffering from a gynaecological cancer, refused all chemotherapy and wept at each consultation, completely unable to speak. The doctors were distraught, for she refused the therapy and antidepressants she was offered. In discussion with her husband, it was discovered that she had been operated on in a private clinic a year earlier, and that the surgeons had promised to follow her up themselves, judging straight away that the situation was not within the remit of a university centre. Unfortunately, unexpected post-operative complications and the departure on holiday of the doctor had necessitated the transfer of the patient to the gynaecological department of a nearby hospital. Following a fresh intervention, she had then been referred for fifteen sessions of radiotherapy. As she had not responded sufficiently to this new treatment, she now found herself in medical oncology, to begin chemotherapy.

This woman, of modest background, expressed herself little and did not have the ability to understand exactly what was happening to her. She had experienced the series of successive interventions as a descent into hell and as abandonment. Passing from the luxurious clinic and the admired doctor to more and more worrying and strange situations had considerably altered her confidence and had panicked her. Finally, the proposal of psychiatric treatment meant for her that there was nothing more to be done. A few sessions of clarification between the patient, her husband, the oncologist and the psychiatrist facilitated an explanation of her state, a sharing of her experience, and a recognition of what had worried her, and enabled sufficiently reassuring solutions to be offered so that finally she was able to accept them. In a short time, the clinical situation improved, for the patient agreed to pursue her treatment, and she was still alive after three years' progress.

The psychological approach to the cancer patient necessitates selective use of the basic elements of psychotherapy: clarification, recommendations, suggestions, work on the context (the spouse, the family, the doctors) but also work at the subjective level of feelings and of certain underlying conflicts.

Among the patients followed during the last few years, a certain number were remarkable for a difficult family history, which complicated their affective and relational life. This suffering hardly surfaced during the telling of their over-rational stories. It seemed to them to be inconceivable to change even a little their attachment to the family system, or to express what some people call their true meaning, the authentic, subjective expression of themselves (Mannoni 1987).

The onset of their cancer seemed to be a kind of response, partially symbolic, to inner and contextual impasses. Cancer would represent a sort of destructive and aggressive compromise between the permanence of respect for parental rules ('I am always loyal . . .') and the pressing need to express oneself, but only in a tolerable form ('I suffer, I have limits because I am ill, and so I can no longer be so devoted'). I believe that this way of expressing oneself through the disease plays a part not only in the phases of stabilization but also in the worsening of the clinical state of patients. It is striking to see that people destroy themselves through disease at a particular moment in their lives. Indeed cancer often arises at a borderline or transitional moment in the existential expectations of patients, above all when their models of relationship with life suffer from a kind of impossibility, a fundamental questioning, and when they feel they have no strength or resources to imagine other solutions. Many people whom I have met were in fact strongly involved in a task devoted to others, an unrealistic enterprise or dream, whether in their family, their work, or above all in their care for others. They also had the characteristic of fearing limitations and conflicts or fearing that things might not follow a certain ideal plan (Guex 1986c). Boszormenyi-Nagy has defined the useful concept of the 'ledger'. This is a certain stock of merit which accumulates in an individual in relation to his family, according to his devotion, what he believes he must sacrifice or give, the way in which he has paid with his person for the well-being of the whole. This ledger is credited with the amounts and values received (Boszormenyi-Nagy and Spark 1973). In general, we all thus gain more or less value, in a given system, which allows us to function in life with a certain autonomy and to express more or less authentically what we are.

In certain difficult situations of life, at the time of stages or conflicts that are hard to overcome, the individual who is objectively entrusted, or who thinks he is entrusted, with the important task of maintaining the happiness or the unity of the group, often to his own detriment, will perhaps be pushed to the extreme limits of his model, or sometimes even reduced to a feeling of utter defeat, in order to accomplish nevertheless a task that has become impossible in his eyes. It is indeed very difficult at times to maintain the unity of a family at the time of certain stages in the life cycle, for example at the time of marriages or deaths. It happens fairly frequently that a person has understood that he had to change something, or to be freed from the usual constraints, by inevitable evolution, as a result of the passing of time or history. It is then that suddenly he will discover that as a reprisal he is deprived of the trust, loyalty, affection or gratification of those around him: rather as if his machine had broken down. Worse, he will often see the collapse of the framework, admittedly repetitive and rigid, which keeps him going but on which his life depends, and which perhaps represents his only wealth but also the only link with a family long dispersed or with which every bond has been broken, but whose function is maintained by the simple need for identity.

In such circumstances, rather in the same way that certain animals go and die, without apparent cause, in response to an ecosystem that escapes us, the 'ledger' may become destructive. It is a way of ending a task and of finally ossifying it, or playing for high stakes rather as suicides do. It is perhaps here, without apparent causal factor, that patients who were thus far hyper-adapted feel this loss of hope and this feeling of abandonment which precede or are close to the appearance of a cancer. Then, at the onset of the cancer, one notes that paradoxically the patients suddenly rediscover their familial role, but now recognizing their new boundaries. This phenomenon is particularly noticeable among women with breast cancer who completely change their role, or similarly, among men going through a crisis at work (Morris *et al.* 1981).

We are also struck by the context in which certain tumours of young adults occur at the age of emancipation. Their disease is devastating, when they are in the process of discovering otherness, love, or the great beyond, and at the same time loyalties, or unfinished business, seem to hold them back in their own family, sometimes wrongly, or to hold them back in the task of maintaining the unity of the family which is not ready to negotiate this important stage of the life cycle. Many experiences correspond to this observation: for example, the young immigrant girl who has just successfully passed her school-leaving examination and is well integrated among the young people of her class. She experiences the sudden onset of ovarian cancer at the time of a school trip and shortly after the divorce of her parents. The parents feel completely isolated without her, for they still speak the language of the country very badly. Father and mother of course meet again at the patient's bedside, in the company of the maternal grandmother, who has received a special visa from her country of origin on compassionate grounds. One might say that everything is normal in this story, but it must be said that in spite of the tragic situation, everyone has the air of being perfectly happy to have come together. And the patient refuses to accept treatment, as if to seal the reunion with her sacrifice. An indication that confirms this is the frequency with which one finds that young cancer patients refuse treatment (Lanski *et al.* 1986). These are often over-responsible adolescents, reasonable, born in families who have delegated to them significant power, but at the price of great dependence on the family circle. It is astonishing to see that this refusal of treatment is often shared by the parents, who argue the case with the doctors. One might therefore say that the disease introduces a kind of change which is actually opposed to change.

Faced with this kind of situation, we favour the re-establishment of a new ledger, in particular when the family is willing to meet with us. It may then be feasible to verbalize what had the function of welding them together, while assessing the balance of things given and received. Another way is to express events in terms of destiny, to retell the history of the family by valuing the wealth of shared experience, clarifying mutual uncertainties, allowing the merits and dues of everyone to be recognized, so as to embark on a common project, with future possibilities, where everyone can find an equal part to play. This work is of course considerable, uncertain, full of pitfalls, but sometimes it allows the development of disease to be suspended, to be given a more favourable turn, and in particular to obtain some surprising remissions, of a kind which cannot always be explained in medical terms (LeShan and Gassman 1958).

When the case can only be handled at an individual level, it is the personal story of people which offers other perspectives, expressed in their choices and their opinions, their humours and their whims, their successes and their setbacks, a sort of balance-sheet capable of guaranteeing the permanent value of what they are.

Case study no. 4

I remember a Czechoslovak colleague, settled for eighteen years in Switzerland, where she had opened a practice. Five years earlier she had married an older divorced man. During the first year of her marriage she had presented with a carcinoma of the cervix, followed several months later by a cancer of the left breast, then, fairly rapidly, a tumour with a different histology in the right breast. At the time of our first interview, she had developed yet another cancer. The patient was overwhelmed, depressed, was having anguished outbursts, and could not be left alone. Her case was undertaken as a matter of urgency, when for the first time the loss of a 'perfect' body and the possibility of decline were recognized. The period was difficult but productive. I discovered that quite recently Mme A. had followed a course of therapy which aimed to reinforce her optimism and the necessity of overcoming everything with objectivity and dynamism, without ever complaining or being depressed at the picture of her life as a whole. She expressed herself in a very rational way, without feeling, as if frozen in an attitude of perfection. She allowed herself no carelessness in her bearing and her remarks. Nevertheless, during the next few weeks things fell into place, and our work centred on the necessity of developing a personal space. From that time appeared interesting developments, to begin with perhaps in the world of objective reality, then more in the subjective sphere. Links could be made between the start of the marriage and the appearance of the cancer. In her work, the patient seemed to know very well how to proceed. Not only was she competent technically, but she organized and directed her relationship with her patients and found pleasure in this, for she was able to devote herself to others, and here applied all the directives received since her childhood. With her husband, on the other hand, she could not assert herself as a doctor (he was not a graduate), which cramped her style and obliged her to adapt to him. She bottled up her feelings, denied her perceptions, and adopted a rigid behaviour, centred mainly on the avoidance of conflict and the search for a harmonious relationship. She had to renounce completely everything that might give her pleasure, in favour of duty. Progressively, she understood that the disease was possibly serving as a protective screen (she could not do everything, take on everything); it was a cry for attention (her husband was made sensitive by the cancer). The creation of an inner space by the disease took the place of the feeling of being bad and inadequate. Further, one had to note that in marrying and allowing herself to experience things for herself, she came into complete contradiction with a certain prohibition hanging over her and a particular relationship with death, as her history demonstrated.

The patient was born in Prague, where her father had died of cancer some time earlier. Her mother, on the point of giving birth, had called a doctor who, judging that labour had not yet started, left her alone. In the morning, he came back and discovered the mother dying. He performed a Caesarian, saving the child *in extremis*. The patient was brought up and exploited by a maternal aunt. She had both to show by brilliant study that she deserved her adoption and at the same time to pay for it by submitting herself to all the humble tasks of the household. Often, when she was not sufficiently obedient, she was threatened with being put in the orphanage. At the same time, it was suggested that she might one day avenge her mother, and medicine was explicitly seen from this viewpoint.

To sum up, one might say that, 'guilty' of being the only survivor of her family, she could only survive effectively in forgetting herself and in devoting herself to others in the hope of total devotion. Being a doctor was to imitate the one who had saved her, but paradoxically it was also to act like the one who had killed her mother, for lack of correct appraisal of the situation. Her fate was then to be irreproachable and faultless, to survive, to correct history, but also so as not to be rejected. To marry, so as to try to live also at an emotional level, completely demolished her system of loyalties. Over several months, I was able to observe a total change in the behaviour of the patient, who set about challenging her husband, made personal demands, and allowed herself periods of relaxation. She travelled, she renegotiated her relationships with her step-family and with her colleagues. Even her appearance changed: from being a rigid person she blossomed, adopted a new hair-style, altered her clothes, and allowed herself to work part-time. Moreover, she dared to affirm her identity as a doctor when she appeared in public, in the company of her husband.

Being able to speak about herself and at the same time change her relationships with others apparently allowed this woman to no longer make herself ill. Unfortunately, she belonged to that category of patients who want the context to be immediately ready to receive them according to their new definition of things, which is seldom possible. And so I was obliged to witness a constant oscillation between the state of illness and that of health in the course of the five years during which our sessions were to last, and this in a way that was totally independent of her chemotherapy treatments. Such therapies are uncertain and long term, where periods of remission alternate with dramatic recurrences, arising every time that the talking therapy or the therapeutic regime does not seem sufficient to guarantee space for thought. At such moments, one might say that the patient cannot resist putting all her energy into mobilizing others (the spouse, the world), even at the price of a relapse. Psychosomatic regression, or recurrence, are then a way of physically putting back into place a system of conditioning, but at the same time of rediscovering the identity of one's roots and family loyalties.

PATIENT GROUPS

One way of helping the patient and his relatives is to form self-help groups, or groups led by professionals – doctors, nurses, or social workers (Ringler *et al.* 1981). In California, around 8,000 patients were involved in such groups in 1983 (Forester *et al.* 1985). This not only seems helpful in maintaining the psychological equilibrium of a large number of people, but also is a way of economizing on scarce resources, if enough trained staff are not available.

Few studies have examined the effect that these groups actually have on patients, with the interesting exception of Spiegel *et al.* (1981, 1989). There are several indications:

- The patients and their families want help in facing up to the emotional impact of cancer, and want more information about treatments.
- Partners want to be involved in the care policy, for they are swamped by emotional reactions that they do not know how to handle.
- Groups often involve relaxation and problem-solving techniques, which are very effective for reducing stress.
- In a group, in the presence of other patients, it is possible to tackle all the practical details of daily life and exchange useful information about the available resources (Spiegel *et al.* 1981).

Whatever the setting adopted (i.e., whether or not members of the health-care team are present), the group not only has a function of information-giving and problem-solving, but it also encourages lively verbal exchanges.

The group members serve as models for each other. In listening to and observing each other, they find a new energy to face up to the situations which they have in common and enhance their adaptative resources. In a word, they help each other, for each one gives and receives at the same time, which reinforces feelings of usefulness and reduces those of powerlessness. The group experience, whether it takes place inside or outside the hospital, facilitates all kinds of adjustments, particularly in reinforcing the sense of community.

Some therapists consider that it must be depressing to meet people who are going through the same tragic experiences. The opinion of the patients is quite different, for they consider the group a privileged place where they can share sometimes morbid fears and pre-occupations, notably anxieties about death. Generally, they cannot do this in their family circle for fear of upsetting and tiring their relatives.

According to Spiegel *et al.* (1981), the experience of altruism is very important. Depressed and hopeless people suddenly discover that they can be useful to others who are even worse off. Moreover, speaking together about hostility and negative feelings is a relief.

Discussing in groups so as to share the distress that is common to all is also a very important aspect, which relieves patients.

Sona Euster, social worker at the Memorial Sloan-Kettering Cancer Center in New York, has well described the groups that she runs for mastectomy patients immediately after their operation:

The Post Mastectomy Rehabilitation Group meets every weekday morning for an hour and a half. Prior to each session, the group leaders confer with nursing staff to exchange information about patients. Their medical situations, physical or emotional prob-lems, and reactions to previous group sessions are discussed, and treatment plans for the group and the hospital unit are formulated. Patients begin to attend the session on the 2nd postoperative day and continue until discharge. Attendance is not mandatory but strongly encouraged by all staff. Introduction of the group and its design are presented by the social worker at each session. Patients are informed of the group structure and its purpose in aiding them with the initial physical and emotional adjustment to mastectomy. Following this, an exercise program is conducted by the physical therapist to aid patients in achieving a normal range of motion in the affected arm. These women have experienced physical losses such as decrease of arm and shoulder function during the initial postoperative stage. . . . This restriction of activity contributes to a sense of helplessness and loss of mastery. The therapist teaches and supervises the execution of five specific exercises, explaining their purpose and importance. After the exercises, Tuesday and Thursday, the nurse informs patients about types of surgical procedures and removal of lymph nodes, and instructs them on the need for hand and arm care, and care of the wound postdischarge. She also provides preliminary information regarding prostheses.

Three times a week, Monday, Wednesday, and Friday, patients participate in a discussion of their concerns and emotional reactions related to the diagnosis of cancer and the surgery.

The group size is 9–12 patients per session, with each patient attending an average of three to four times prior to discharge. Each day new patients may attend and others may be discharged. The daily repetition of the exercises serves a double purpose: It provides patients with an opportunity to complete one of five exercise sessions prescribed per day, and it enables them to begin the work of developing trust and group cohesion. By working together on a physical activity, patients meet one another and begin to recognize commonalities in their situations. They begin to know one another through a shared mutual task. Since this is an open-ended group, there is a continual need for emotionally safe common ground for the initiation of group process. The exercises provide this.

Repetition of the nursing information twice weekly and alternation of this with the discussion periods contribute to a unique meshing of facts and feelings, each enhancing the other. . . . These discussion sessions, approximately 45 minutes in length, are conducted by the social worker with the assistance of a Reach to Recovery volunteer. Reach to Recovery is a branch of the American Cancer Society consisting of trained volunteers who have previously undergone mastectomies.

(Euster 1979: 256–7)

The volunteer is called on to offer honest reassurance and not to idealize her experience. She deals with both negative and positive aspects of her story, and she therefore shows patients that it is possible to overcome mutilation and even to succeed in resuming a satisfying life. In hearing this life-story, patients are encouraged to speak similarly about themselves. The role of social worker is to facilitate the expression and control of feelings.

The group allows us to recognize the universality of the questions that are asked and the reactions that arise. It is above all centred on comparison, personal interaction, and abreaction, which are indispensable factors in overcoming crises. This model is not solely applicable to women who have undergone mastectomies but can be extended to all categories of cancer patients. It is not necessary to recruit exclusively people suffering from the same pathology; sometimes the mix of different experiences turns out to be even more helpful.

COGNITIVE-BEHAVIOURAL METHODS

Cognitive-behavioural methods are of special interest when attempting to remedy the practical problems arising from cancer and its treatments. In recent years many studies have attempted to describe the techniques that are helpful in reducing the psychosomatic symptoms and the side-effects of treatments among both children and adults. There is no question of replacing individual psychotherapy; it is simply a supplementary contribution to the usual methods. In fact, the goal is not to work on psychological conflicts or defences but to attempt a relatively direct modification of maladaptive or reactive behaviour:

– an attempt to correct definite and well-defined symptoms;
– the technique to take account of the experience and the wishes of the patient;
– a time-limited intervention;
– a method that is assessable in terms of the patient's behavioural change;
– with the possibility of interrupting, continuing, or changing the strategy according to the patient's response.

Certain patients are extremely resistant to the idea of speaking about their lives and their psychological problems. On the other hand, they are attracted if one proposes a technique that seeks to resolve their problems in a concrete way. Another advantage lies in the fact that the strategies used, which are short term and centred on the problems of cancer. resemble the other types of therapeutic management and are therefore very well accepted and understood by other cancer specialists. It is a relatively new field, and the clinical studies on this subject are rare or still incomplete (Burish and Lyles 1979; Greer et al. 1992).

It has been observed that on top of the nausea and vomiting caused by chemotherapy, 25 per cent of patients developed anticipatory side-effects, and that this was a matter of acquired behaviour (Redd et al. 1982a). It is for this type of problem, as also for chronic pain, that cognitive-behavioural methods have been shown to be the most effective.

The technique is a hypnotic procedure induced by the therapist, who teaches the patient muscular relaxation and guided imagery. Certain patients may be afraid of the idea of undergoing 'hypnosis', but this reluctance seems to be linked with the word rather than the

technique (Sacerdote 1966). 'Hypnotherapy' may be a more acceptable term which is widely used.

When the patient is seated on a comfortable chair, or lying on a
bed, the therapist asks him to focus on a point in the room. He then
suggests to the patient that he concentrate his attention on the
sensations which he feels in the various muscle groups. He then
suggests the progressive extension of relaxation to other areas, until
complete bodily comfort is obtained. Another method is to begin
with breathing, as in yoga. At each inhalation, the patient is
encouraged to feel his inner space opening up and also his capacity
for containment, which sets the boundaries of the external world.
Each exhalation is associated with the loosening of the chest and
abdominal muscles, the lowering of the shoulders and the descent
into an even deeper state of relaxation.

When the patient is calm and still, the therapist suggests to him
pleasant and soothing images, which are either linked with his past
or, failing that, scenes that are generally appreciated by everybody,
like the water of a lake, the beach, the freshness of spring, warm
sand, the breeze. If a patient particularly likes a personal scene, he is
encouraged to make use of it. One can add to this a correlation with
other sensory systems, suggesting that he should imagine the different colours of the rainbow (passing from the deep and stimulating
colours towards ever paler and more serene colours) or sinking still
deeper into the chair with every exhalation. Following the sensory
manner of functioning preferred by the patient, who perhaps is not
particularly visual but more sensitive to sounds or to smells, it is
possible to add other synaesthetic modalities – a familiar tune, a
sensation of cold or warmth, a position, or a scent.

It is necessary to try two or three exercises of this kind before
using them during chemotherapy. If the symptoms of nausea appear
all the same, the therapist takes up the images that have been used
previously, filling in more details and amplifying them. The basic
strategy is to turn the attention away and to check carefully the
reactions or the indirect messages given by the patient, so as to be
able to modify his perceptions. The patient must always be allowed
to choose, so that he feels free. If he wants to open his eyes or come
out of his state of trance for a moment, this must be accepted, for the
splitting up of the operation has a reinforcing effect. If the patient
collaborates, things go well. For some patients, the symptoms return
if the therapist is not there; in this case the exercise must be repeated.

The method is equally effective for controlling patients' fears and pain, when anxiolytics and analgesics are insufficient. It has great value for reducing stress. It is possible to elaborate the exercise by proposing to the patient when in trance that he should confront anxiogenic situations. He is thus able, in a protective and secure framework, as an exercise, to review his various strengths and choose the best one to confront what stresses him.

In surgery, hypnotic procedures may enable the pain of certain techniques to be avoided, such as the insertion of a nasogastric feeding tube in the case of vomiting. The hypnotic induction of local anaesthesia in people who are allergic to injections is also helpful.

According to the degree of seriousness of the illness and their physical state, patients feel extremely devalued, no longer being able to trust their body, whose image is so much changed. It then happens that they focus everything on the external world, which they expect to provide magical assistance, often in an aggressive manner. The relaxation associated with a positive visualization of the intact areas of the body, starting from which a certain control may be exercised by the mind on the diseased areas, allows the cancer patient to reduce his sensitivity to the external world and to make a peaceful return into himself, especially if he is helped to do this (Simonton *et al.* 1978).

Cognitive-behavioural intervention is not merely a manipulatory technique, but it is also an alliance and an active collaboration between patient and therapist, who are working towards a precise goal. If the envisaged results come about, this is a factor in the opening-up of a relationship of trust that can finally lead to psychotherapeutic work.

Case study no. 5

A young father developed an aggressive melanoma in multiple sites, creating a serious risk of death from haemorrhage. He refused to see his wife and children and maintained a hostile attitude towards the team, for he reckoned he had been put in an inferior room, with a disagreeable neighbour in the next bed. It was obvious that this man was extremely traumatized and distressed, made a total abstraction of his body, and found no respite to reflect and put his affairs in order so as to best employ the remaining time left to him. All verbal approaches were refused. It was suggested that he should try a technique for the better control of his tension and distress. In fact, in the course of a relaxation, he found comfort for the first time in ages and allowed his thoughts and his emotions to be directed towards peaceful and reassuring scenes. Repeating the exercise daily, he progressively took over a certain control of the situation. He was then able to discuss together with his wife and the therapist and decide on his next return home, and to define the conditions. Then he consented to see his children, even to spend time with them and broach with them certain plans of concern to them.

BODY WORK

At Lausanne, the technique used is essentially based on the eutony of Gerda Alexander (1971), already widely tested in occupational therapy with many groups of psychosomatic patients. Elements of Schulz's autogenic training are also combined with it, and the massage and manipulation used in physiotherapy. The aim is to help patients who have been assaulted by the disease and the treatments to create for themselves a peaceful personal space and to reconcile themselves with this body which has betrayed them.

Eutony integrates the concepts of 'body unity', 'contact', and 'movement in space'; these are the elements that can be utilized in the different exercises, which can be done individually, in pairs, or as a group (Vayer 1973; Pasini and Andreoli 1981).

Often, for the cancer patient, the body is felt to be fragmented. It is therefore helpful to work on reconstructing somatic unity through the perception of the patient and the definition that he is able to make of himself in space and time. Relaxation exercises enable him to discover in his body a possible source of well-being through warmth, calm and security; he regains body awareness and discovers that it is part of his personal unity and thus of his capacity to define himself in relation to the external world.

The exercises are done by using objects (stick, balloon, roll or cushion), by massage and direct contact, and by passive manipulation. Some work is done on the refinement of the patient's perception, which reinforces body awareness and facilitates the development of a feeling of inner security. In this way the patient learns to control his body and make of it once more a powerful ally. According to the areas of the body which he is working on – for example, lying on his back, making a rotatory movement, or observing the breaking down into its component parts of a movement that is usually automatic – the patient will learn to discriminate better between pleasant and unpleasant sensations and to master certain pains, which is essential to the rediscovery of a certain well-being. It is not a question of regressing to a primitive stage of instinctive security, but rather of embarking on the personal enterprise of putting one's body in working order. A better perception of one's body and its limits facilitates the widening of the areas of exchange with the outside world, which helps the ability to adapt and to react to events. This is a way not only of becoming familiar with the body (often ruled out by the illness), but also of reclaiming it and preserving it as a constituent element of one's personality and identity. The patient then seems better equipped to overcome the existential breakup which he is experiencing, and to retain a certain control.

Certain other techniques develop the consciousness of the body's shape and spatial limits. Such are, for example, exercises in touching. The skin is the organ which envelops the body and delimits it, while being the interface with the context. For example, the awareness of touching the ground with the soles of the feet in a vertical position, or the legs, back, arms, and head in a lying position, or of the parts in contact with a chair, facilitates the development of postural consciousness. Working on certain particular areas, or focusing exclusively on parts that are intact, allows the patient to turn away from his diseased area and to discover in his body not only a place of retreat but also a multitude of possibilities of contact with the other.

Movements in space complete such approaches. They facilitate the perception of a continuity between inner body space and external space. The patient can learn to play with the alternation of tension and relaxation, of opening out and of withdrawing into himself; this is the revaluing of personal rhythm as opposed to the tempo imposed by the medical set-up. The adequate execution of a movement, or of any activity, implies at the same time an awareness of the movement itself, of the space in which it is practised and of the most appropriate rhythm for doing it. Here are the means that serve to seek or rediscover a certain psychosomatic balance, and by extension to become aware, or to keep one's distance, in relation to the significant discrepancy between the artificial rhythm imposed on the body by the outside world and its own biological rhythm. This is a way of combating stress effectively.

These exercises and methods are usually practised in small groups; this offers the same advantages as those described in the section above dealing with patient groups (Guex and MacDonald 1984).

Chapter 13

Terminal illness

GENERAL

It is essential that at the end of his life the patient should benefit from the same attention as at the moment of diagnosis and during his treatment. It is not simply a question of offering him physical and moral support, but also of giving him the chance to develop as far as possible the potential for life which remains to him, in terms of activity, creativity and human relationships.

According to Cecily Saunders, pioneer of the hospice movement in Great Britain, terminal care 'refers to the management of patients in whom the advent of death is felt to be certain and not too far off and for whom medical effort has been turned away from [active] therapy and become concentrated on the relief of symptoms and the support of both patient and family' (Holford 1972 quoted in Saunders 1982). As the terminal phase may last for some time, it requires much flexibility, initiative and skill on the part of carers (Saunders 1982).

Physical comfort means above all relief from pain, which has been discussed earlier, and, of course, freedom from a wide range of symptoms which require a textbook on internal medicine: anorexia, digestive problems, dyspnoea, incontinence and urinary retention, pruritus, sore mouth. Psychological disorders are also frequent, such as anxiety and depression, insomnia, confusion or agitation (Mosley 1985).

Doctors should give the appropriate care at each stage of the illness, but without being limited only to technical interventions. The aim is not to prolong life, but to relieve suffering. Too often, the problems of euthanasia and suicide arise when patients experience too great pain and serious concerns that are not dealt with. These ethical questions can only find answers, in any case, by analysing the context of each individual situation. Thus, for each treatment, the risks, the pain, the chance of success, the anticipated results, and the side-effects must be carefully assessed. It is easier to be prudent and forgo some treatment rather than have to interrupt it when it has already been established. The patient, if possible, but also the family must be partners in the decision-making process, and it is always necessary to clarify with them the chosen course of action. It sometimes happens that some patients want to resume a more aggressive or active treatment. The general rule is then to maintain a certain flexibility and, instead of following rigid procedures, it is better to feel one's way and discuss so as to verify whether the chosen path is always the best. This way of approaching the patient in the terminal phase offers a form of 'creativity' which preserves the patient's value and supports him in his feelings.

DOMICILIARY CARE AND THE HOSPICE CONCEPT

During the past decade a great effort has been made to promote the well-being of the dying, and issues such as 'death with dignity', the 'right to die' and the 'rights of the dying' have been addressed with clarity. The principle of the 'good death' has given rise to the hospice movement, pioneered by St Christopher's in London (Krant *et al.* 1976; Leone 1982; Saunders 1982).

When the decision has been taken to stop treatment, many questions arise: What to say to the patient? Who will speak to him? How will the family members react? How will this family be involved in care? What procedure should be introduced for the preparation for death? Will the patient remain at home, will he go into a hospice (if one exists in the area), or will he be hospitalized? What are the out-patient facilities available? Who will support the team or the family? What role will the doctor continue to play (Christensen and Harding 1985)? Replies to these questions should be clarified and conscientiously negotiated in each case. Nonetheless, certain broad principles may be set out: the integration of support services, the maintenance of stability, and getting the best value from the time that remains (Kübler-Ross 1969, 1978).

The cornerstone of all intervention is the maintenance of the relationship that has been established with the treating physician, who knows his patient and his clinical state and should take an active part in management. The patient cannot bear it if his doctor withdraws, and his presence, even without treatment, guarantees the continuance of a certain hope. After having accepted the inevitable approach of his death, the patient may continue to think of his doctor as his sole link with a viable future.

If possible, the patient should not be subjected to a complete upheaval and change of surroundings, whether of his usual environment or of the team that has so far managed his case and with which significant relationships have developed (nurse, social worker, or clergy). After all, it is with the team that 90 per cent of the duration of the illness has been shared. Maintaining a certain continuity of care, without dramatic change, allows the maximum moral and emotional support to be offered. Every effort should be made by the services concerned to ensure that the patient may remain at home, by organizing the appropriate care in co-operation with the family. This may last for several weeks or several months, and when things have been well planned, most families accept death at home, for they feel supported.

If home care remains the exception, perhaps this is a result, during recent years, of the technological development of medicine, particularly in the hospital setting, of a lack of information on the availability of domiciliary help, or of the decline in the practice of visiting; but still more often, doctors neglect or are ignorant of the possibility of correct treatment at home. In the United States, except for certain sophisticated procedures, everything can be done in the patient's home: medical visits, nursing care, occupational therapy, hiring of auxiliary equipment, and other technical services such as inserting catheters or drips for ensuring bodily functions or pain relief (Koren 1986).

The last aspect, 'enriching the time that remains', was admirably illustrated by Elisabeth Kübler-Ross in her book *To live until we say good-bye*:

Our role in their struggle was simply as a catalyst, to share a moment, a tear perhaps, a hope, and most of all, to lend a listening ear. Each one in his or her own private, intimate way had choreographed his or her own death; all were convinced about their own ultimate destiny and had made their own arrangements in keeping with the style of their personality, in style with their character. Each one chose to live to the very end in the way he or she found to be most meaningful. . . . [P]erhaps it will help you, if nothing else, to share the deepest thoughts and dreams of others

who have preceded you in death and somehow have shown you the
way it can be for you if you choose to have it that way. . . .

(Kübler-Ross 1978: 13–14)

This approach recognizes the patient's needs and mobilizes all the
available resources that can be helpful to him. Since dying is the last
stage of life, most people manage to concentrate their thoughts on the
quality of life, even at the final moment, if they are helped to do this.
This is why efforts should be centred on the enrichment of the time
that remains. The family, friends and health professionals must be
shown that they can play an active part in this.

The work which is done at the Victoria Hospital in Montreal is
important in this respect. Patients in this hospital who are at the
terminal stage are integrated with chronic patients who must learn to
live from day to day. Thus time is broken up and valued, so as to make
a defence against death. The original element is that teams favour the
re-establishment of familiar rituals, that is to say, the representation
of the dialogue between life and death by songs, games or other group
activities. Each benefits moreover from a special relationship with a
nurse, with whom he can speak of his concerns. An important place is
given to families, who feel welcome, are integrated with the team,
and stay in the hospital with their relatives. Within the limits of the
possible, everything is said about the state of being seriously ill, and
equally, everything is done to protect the group and the survivors, and
death comes gently (Mount 1980).

SUPPORTING THE PATIENT

When we speak of supporting and partnering the patient, we often
insist on practical and technical arrangements that must be borne in
mind. The doctor or the health-care teams find it difficult to admit
that comfort, or a deeper understanding of the patient's needs, can be
effective responses to the terminal situation. In their eyes, this is an
'esoteric', displaced attitude, producing anxiety or wasting time. The
most widespread idea is that one should not confront somebody who
is already seriously ill with further psychological conflicts, which
may seriously upset a fragile equilibrium. But, unlike many
psychiatric patients who resist their doctors' interpretations, the
cancer patient, beginning the final phase of his life, is very often
anxious to speak of the meaning of his life or of his behaviour
(Verwoerdt 1966).

In the classical models of treatment, medical information is usually given, illustrated by statistical predictions, and the history of the disease precedes that of the patient, independently of it. Death is already written in the text, before being so in the heart. In the course of months, through his need to be helped and to calm his distress, the patient has been subjected to this new technical perspective and will have forgotten what gave him his own direction, his experience, his personal history, his life. Support will have as its first function to re-create this space, where the dying person becomes again a living person who is going to die. This move may be called 'speaking to oneself'; that is, in the words of Michel de Certeau (1975), 'between the machine which stops or breaks down, and the act of dying, there is the possibility of saying it. The "dying" takes place between the two.' Being able to speak of oneself is perhaps a sacred act. The sacred is, indeed, an element determining the awareness by man of his being as man, which is something other than a simple human being expecting to survive physically. In extreme situations, man finds himself in a universe which is altogether too much for him. The need for dialogue, the quest for meaning, and the emergence of spiritual needs are perhaps the only ways of getting through this phase, by escaping destructive destiny and putting oneself in the position of a being relinked with others by communication, meditation or prayer (Frankl 1962; de M'Uzan 1981).

Case study no. 6

Mme S., an expatriate, had only seen her family once in six years, at the funeral service of her older sister, who had died of cancer. Being herself at an advanced stage of her own cancer, she longed to understand her illness, and even at this point, to settle her position with her family. She wanted to know if what had happened to her had a link with what she had experienced with her relations. Three years earlier she had married a divorced man, the father of a little girl of 10. It was at the time that she ardently wished for a child that the first symptoms of the disease became evident. How to interpret her wish to understand? Was this a flight from reality, that is to say, death, a displacement of the problem, or on the other hand the need to mobilize her family at a tragic moment? It was certain that she was determined to fight right to the end, with all her strength.

The situation seemed fairly tense with her husband, who was devoted to her but by whom she did not feel understood. She was used to caring for others rather than herself; her late marriage to a man with certain problems was a demonstration of this. She had difficulty in expressing her feelings, her anger or her anxiety, and systematically avoided conflict, taking refuge behind a calm and serene façade. She still allayed suspicion extremely well, and this frame of mind enabled her to maintain a pleasant relationship with her doctors. Contacts were warm and dynamic during consultations, but she felt completely abandoned between times. She suffered more and more loss of control over daily life and her physical functions, and saw herself progressively sinking into social and emotional isolation.

I understood her situation, but it was difficult for me, in such a context, to speak with her only about her family, for the priority was to re-evaluate the conditions of her well-being and envisage a global management. To help her in her feeling of abandonment and despair, it was necessary to form a sort of substitute family: friends were recruited to take turns at her bedside; a home help took care of the housework and the cooking; finally, the doctors promised to change their way of communicating with her and to improve her physical comfort.

The first stage was then to clarify with the patient what family she had need of; perhaps it was a question here of a therapeutic family and of arranging proper help at home. The second stage was certainly to work with the real family, in this case the husband, to enable him to speak of his feelings in the face of an overwhelming fate and to help him to improve communications with his wife. While taking account of their personalities, I tried to establish how the husband could help the patient directly, in cosseting her, touching her, or quite simply holding her hand to listen to her. It was then that she was able, in her turn, to begin to express her guilt and to speak of her worthlessness, her fear of not being up to her husband's expectations.

This focusing brought about an astonishing subjective improvement in the patient; in fact, she was able to get up little by little, to take care of herself to some extent and to regain some strength. But there remained for her a great concern, that of maintaining a satisfactory self-image, of bolstering her self-esteem. She was very coquettish and took the devastatation of the disease badly; she wished moreover to be more active at home, and she had to find ways of regaining some control over her body. I undertook twice-weekly sessions of relaxation with positive visualization of the body, with the help of pictures, stories and travel, which had been her greatest pleasures at all periods of her life. This enabled her to feel better and put her in touch with herself. After a certain time, she dared to swim every day in the swimming-pool of her block of flats when nobody was around. She was delighted with this improvement in the quality of her life. This work offered her more inner security, and she could then speak of her anguish at having broken with her roots and transgressed the rules of her family by marrying a divorced man. She could even give meaning to her illness, which in her eyes protected her from the feeling of being a bad girl. This was when she began to speak of her people and of the nostalgia which linked her with her far-off origins. She had broken with her country ten years before, and for the whole of this time she had struggled against unresolved 'bad' feelings in herself while she fled around the world.

Born in a German family of small farmers, austere Protestants, she was the second in a family of seven. The father devoted himself to work and the mother looked after everything else, continually exhausted. Sometimes, the mother came to admit that life was hard, but reckoned that it was impossible to escape her fate. In the eyes of Mme S., her elder sister had acquired a particular status, having the right to flout a very rigid moral code, but she had perhaps died because of this. The patient had long adopted a different position, taking on her responsibilities, but without ever heeding her desires or acknowledging what she felt deeply. She was completely devoted and submissive to the family norms. Up till the age of 20, she had not gone out but looked after her brothers and sisters, without being able to protect her personal space. When she rebelled a little, she felt immediately denigrated by her mother. She said, 'They always overworked me; I questioned the system, but I could never speak up for myself; I think they never loved me.' It was only as an adult that she left her family to become a nurse, never to return.

It was from this stage that it was possible to sort out her loyalties with regard to her relatives. Perhaps feeling bad was reinforced by the fact that she had abandoned her family and her central role as 'parentified' child. So as to maintain her debts intact, she had decided, originally, to live abroad – an apparent emancipation – but sacrificing herself as a nurse and staying celibate. She had then taken on the role of her dead sister, just after having discovered the 'egoistic' happiness of marriage.

Once she had been able to achieve this new assessment, she asked her family to come and see her. They all came together around her bed, when she came to be hospitalized, and it was there that, rather than speaking about everything, they were at least able to touch and hug each other.

Case study no. 7

Mlle S., 40 years old, a teacher, suffered from a gastric cancer; at the point of death, she asked for a consultation, because she was very anxious about her mother, who just had an operation for breast cancer. She was extremely jaundiced, and was dozing in her bed. She spoke of herself, of her feeling of dying at the moment when she had at last found her vocation. In fact, as the eldest of a family of three daughters, she had always been the favourite companion of the father, an intellectual who did not express his feelings. She was a brilliant student of linguistics and formal logic, seeking above all to dissect and understand the mysteries of existence. Her emotional life had been fairly impoverished, marked by a single affair with a mathematician, in every respect similar to her father. Five years earlier, she had broken off this relationship, for she felt bound to suppress her own feelings in order to protect her friend's pride.

In spite of the fact that her days were numbered and that she knew it, this patient was very keen to understand why she was sacrificing herself once again in dying. It seemed clear that she had been in the grip of a crisis of identity and of role. She oscillated between the desire to please her father and so to live in disembodied celibacy, and that of allowing herself to follow her feelings as a woman and to resemble her mother, who was crushed.

A short time after having broken off her relationship, she enrolled in music courses at the conservatoire; at the time that her cancer was discovered, she had become a soloist in a choir. Her last years had been a time of intense pleasure, with the impression that she was at last finding herself. For a week, we spoke of her guilt towards her parents; she reproached herself for being unable to help them on the threshold of old age, and this tormented her a great deal. We made an assessment of what she had brought to them (being a companion to the father, so as to support the mother), and of what she had received (a broad culture and great intellectual capacity). In running through all this, it became clearly apparent to her that she had done enough. The role of the therapist (in the place of the parents, who were too involved in their own problems) was to give her permission to live her own life, and to make the most of the time that remained to her.

And so we planned relaxation sessions, with guided imagery, to help her to experience as comfortably as possible – and according to her own system of representation – the long hours passed alone in her room. We said goodbye the evening before a weekend during which she died, apparently serene.

In the two preceding examples, we have seen that specific understanding of the individual needs, emotions, and concerns of the patient, to which one must know how to tune in, offers a guide to choosing the most helpful approach. The first patient spontaneously consulted her family, from which arose the problem of isolation when faced with the group. To help her meant to redefine the policy of home care and her place in relation to others. The second patient spoke rather of her identity and of her creativity. She had a strong wish to live as far as possible 'egoistically' during her last hours (Guex 1982). In the following example, the patient made a request for psychotherapy.

Case study no. 8

Mme A. was born in Switzerland, in the country. She had a younger brother and sister, who had completed courses of study and married. The father, 70 years old, was a weak person who protected himself behind a wall of aggressiveness and rigidity. He seemed unhappy, hardly able to bear vexation. The mother, aged 60, appeared self-effacing, resigned, and mistrustful of her daughter, with whom she would have no dealings until she had to care for her when the illness took a turn for the worse.

The patient had little affinity with her younger brother and sister. She could not recall any discussion within the family, where feelings were rarely expressed. She thought she was like her father, but she had never been able to develop her relationship with him because of the hostile attitude which he adopted, and above all for fear of 'betraying' her mother, the powerless victim. She reckoned to have scarcely ever had the leisure to think of herself. As a child, she dreamt of the way in which she would lead her life when she was free of all these family shackles. After a problem-free school career, and in spite of her wish to take up fine art, she took a rapid secretarial course and spread her wings. She rushed into marriage with an older man by whom she had two children. She hardly spoke of this conjugal relationship, except to say that there was no conflict there.

The only details that she volunteered concerned her sense of duty, the desire that everyone around her should be happy, and her general impression of having accomplished her task as wife and mother as well as possible.

Attacked by a metastatic cancer which was resistant to treatment, she asked to see the psychiatrist, wishing to 'live her death'. The interviews took place at her home for two months, twice a week at the end of the day, in the room where she had to stay in bed. Her contact with the outside world was provided for by the visits of her relations and the home helps. She spoke with them quite freely about her cancer, in a realistic manner, and without any affectation, as if to keep her position of amenable mother-wife-patient who wants to take up the least possible room and allow others to get on with their lives as if nothing were amiss.

Once the door of her room was shut, during these interviews, the patient allowed herself an outburst of anguish and rage. Rage against herself, for having succumbed, but also rage against the others, the doctors, to whom she partly attributed her defeat. On some occasions, she was so tense that this prevented her from breathing and from drinking; at such times, she froze in her bed and gazed fixedly at the wall.

Our common task consisted in preparing the patient to face death. And so we decided to go on meeting until the end, in a relationship where the doctor would be the neutral and benevolent witness of the formation of a 'creative process', aimed at allowing the patient to say or find out who she was. It seems that this woman, who had never known or been able to clarify what she was, was now, thanks to the progression of the cancer, setting about expressing herself and saying 'I'.

In a very distressing atmosphere, it all began with a minute description of her visualization of this thing within her, compressing the healthy organs. Taming the cancer was the point of departure for a new drama in which we were the actors. At times, the description of the tumour was dissociated from her emotions, and we could then speak of the disease as of a third party, of which I sometimes had to become the protagonist, for she questioned me about my own possible death from cancer. I had the impression of entering into a new world whose limits are blurred, whose identities are uncertain. At the end of certain sessions, going down the stairs in her house, I wondered why I was not myself dying. We often spoke of quite different things, and particularly of her plans stimulated by the view from her window of flowering springtime. These were the first poetic elements of her vocabulary, which enabled her to give free rein to her imagination. Thus, she evoked for the first time the period of her childhood with her parents in the country. This alternation between plain description of the clinical reality and making calm plans, this active struggle against the fragmentation of the cancer, made possible the birth of an imaginary space of which she seemed to have been bereft up till now.

At the end of some weeks, she succeeded in letting herself go a little; I found her more relaxed, often dozing on her bed, making no complaint. Sometimes, she spontaneously recounted her daydreams: a temple in Tibet, where she gave herself to meditation and creation. At other times, she told me about her dreams where she saw herself in dialogue with someone very close, perhaps her double, that part of herself as a little girl that she had forgotten on the way, full of feelings and of hope. She also spoke to me of my work, of my accompaniment of cancer patients, as if by this I also stood for this double in some way, this part that was ejected from herself with the cancer, which would perhaps survive her, marked with her imprint, or which would die in her place, as if she were no more concerned by this huge problem.

One day, feeling my presence in her room, she asked me to keep silent, for fear that I would bring her back to the bank. She was on a boat that was floating away, and I only held the end of a long rope. It was at this time that she spontaneously re-established contact with her mother, with whom she began to spend long hours without talking, simply appreciating the pleasure and the warmth of her touch. This return of the mother corresponded to her dreams, whose dominant theme was the sea or the oceans to be crossed to reach the antipodes, in other words, the voyage.

One evening, she declared that she felt near the end, and that it seemed important to speak with her people. I therefore went to find them, and retired. The next day, she passed away.

SUPPORT BY THE CARERS

It is not always possible to be attentive to the deep processes of patients or to analyse systematically the models of communication and the types of relationships established by the members of the family. Sometimes, time, availability, interest or competence is lacking. Nevertheless, contact and dialogue with a patient, which are the basis of every relationship, cannot be made in a casual way. The manner of approaching the subject plays a definitive part in helping the dying. Certain points of reference should be respected in order to set up a framework. To be ready to listen means to have a certain capacity for empathy (Tyner 1985). Empathy is not only an inner attitude or a personal aptitude, but also a capacity to behave in such a way that the client feels that he is understood. In other words, it is a process that occurs at the level of the imagination and of behaviour, which Tyner (following Buber 1937 and Reik 1948) has analysed well:

- the capacity for identifying with the patient and for showing that one shares his experience;
- taking into account this shared experience, allowing the social distance to be reduced;
- immediacy, or 'reverberation': reflecting back what one has understood, by formulating it in terms of personal experience (for example saying 'I too feel in a difficult situation in relation to you'); and
- finally, detachment, or establishing a certain distance so as to find an 'objectivity' and equilibrium and so to relieve the feeling of tension.

Kübler-Ross (1978), for example, communicates, by her attitude and her behaviour, the authentic effort which she makes to go to meet the unique experience, past and present, of the person she accompanies. It is in perceiving this effort that the patient can feel himself understood.

Most empathic attitudes are non-verbal: gestures, looks, body language. To stimulate the patient in a tactile way, to touch him, augments this ability to communicate (McCorkle 1974). To sit beside the bed, without saying anything, simply putting a hand on his arm, may be a good way of beginning at the time of a first encounter, after being introduced and saying why one is there.

One cannot foresee everything. One must judge 'instinctively' whether it is better to stay silent, to speak, or to withdraw a little, when one has the impression that the patient and his family are not yet ready to share their suffering.

According to Carkhuff (1969), the patient who asks for help expects complete attention, a realistic attitude, honesty and trust, a good control of the interpersonal distance, and an absence of value-judgement. Probably no help is possible without empathy, that is, without understanding what the patient himself understands. This is the basis of the relational process, which gives value to the messages that are given and received.

People in this situation are confronted by important problems of change. Patients and families have need of help to face up to the changes that correspond with the stages of the disease. There is a long series of new situations which demand practical solutions and, every time, emotional adaptation. Perhaps at the beginning the patient is still autonomous and can express his way of seeing things; he can easily make his wishes known. Further on, while he still makes his presence fully felt, he no longer manages to respond to certain expectations or to take decisions. If it is not understood that he is no longer able to choose, or no longer has the strength, the most simple gestures can be the object of endless prevarication. The relatives, used to react for many years according to a certain perception of things, suddenly have to understand all at once that decisions now depend only on them. It is the job of the health-care team, thanks to their external position, to appreciate these moments and to be generous with sensible advice. To be able to say things and redefine roles often eases tensions and fears and allows the re-establishment of a certain security (Goland 1981).

The principle, then, is to tailor care to the individual and to be available when needed. Things must be analysed according to the strengths and weaknesses of the available resources, for example, establishing who is strong enough to take a turn at the bedside, and so on. The 'harvest of data' is obtained by observation, information, exchange and comparison with past experiences. One of the first assessments to make is to define the expectations and goals of the people one is dealing with, and what may be the means they have at their disposal to attain them.

The general framework of an intervention might be defined in the following way:

- Provision of opportunity for the persons involved to 'tell the story'
- Recognition and acceptance of the varied emotions that people express in relation to a significant loss
- Provision of support for the expression of difficult feelings, such as anger and sadness, with a recognition that people have to do this in their own way and in their own time frame
- Inclusion of children in the grieving process
- Encouragement in the maintenance of established relationships

– Acknowledgement of the usefulness of mutual help groups
– Encouragement of self-care by family members, with particular attention to the person who is the primary caregiver
– Acknowledgement of the usefulness of counseling for problems that seem especially difficult.

(Benoliel 1985: 445, following Bristor 1984)

These principles also aim to protect people from isolation (Zack 1985). The dying person and his family in fact combine all the conditions conducive to the experience of loneliness. Often, the instinctive action to assuage emotional suffering is to isolate oneself (I am thinking particularly of a young patient who completely turned away from his sister, even though he adored her, because she had just had a child, with potential for life, while he himself was preparing to die; this sister had moreover named her son after her sick brother). It thus happens that the dying person breaks essential bonds so as to ensure his short-term comfort, but in this way cuts himself off from very enriching emotional resources which might sustain him for longer. Sometimes we have to note this kind of decision, but then foresee substitute structures, by mobilizing other relatives, other visitors (volunteers, clergy, psychologists) or by steering the patient towards certain practical activities. Sometimes, the patient renounces not only very significant people, but also activities that are very important for him, so as not to suffer any nostalgia and to avoid being confronted by a lessening of his performance. It is possible to channel the energy thus made available into new things which have a similar function. In this way, Elisabeth Kübler-Ross encourages her patients to paint, draw, write or weave rather than wait for hypothetical visits from their children.

It is clear that under this whole philosophy of care lies the problem of loss and grief. The preparation for death, whether for the patient himself or for his relatives, means above all the acceptance of a certain number of losses, whether of persons or of things which gave meaning to the individual's life. Loss is a central experience of human destiny, and people have very variable ways of adapting to it. It will, of course, depend on personal and social resources, on existing affective bonds, but equally on previous experiences and on the availability or otherwise of a protective environment (Benoliel 1985). It is not unusual that loss threatens personal integrity, for a whole life may revolve around one person or one activity. One often has the impression that it is rather the loss of the meaning of life than the loss of the object itself which is then important (Fortini and Wyss 1985; Crisp 1986).

THE SPIRITUAL NEEDS OF THE DYING; SUPPORT BY THE CLERGY

Everything that I have been able to say in this book about the accompaniment of cancer patients concerns not only support and the organization of appropriate care, but even more the respect and the valuing, as much for them as for us, the care-givers, of a history, of an awareness – in a word, of an inwardness.

The preparation for death 'actually goes beyond death, to focus on the consciousness of mortality, or the other side of dying', whether from a secular 'philosophical' perspective or a religious one. Even people who are the most resistant to the transcendental dimension of the human being know that 'the singular being that inhabits the body is not extinguished in the bodily existence, however multiple and intimate the bodily activity may be' (Tilliette 1985).

Rather prosaically, it might be said that, even if the individual has no faith in a revelation, he has the essential need to grant himself in imagination a delay of his own execution; as it is impossible to imagine himself dead, this is a way of gaining a little immortality, and above all of not feeling alone, completely cut off from other human beings.

Care-givers, and particularly doctors, are generally very ill at ease when patients speak of their spiritual needs and question them about their own beliefs. This unease is as great as when it is a matter of death itself, as if one were always confronted here by something indecent. For us, of course, it is clearly a confrontation, as in a mirror, and so a calling into question of our own spiritual pre-paredness.

The secret is not to know everything, or to have ready-made replies, but simply to put up with being a listener, even a silent and powerless one. If this fails, dialogue risks spoiling the opportunity for a unique and exceptional exchange, and by an imperceptible shift, slips into the standard formula where the one suffers and the other treats.

The carer must be able to go beyond this conflict between the secular and the religious, accepting that it is a matter of the search for meaning (Frankl 1962). At these moments, the help of a chaplain (of the appropriate faith) may be invaluable, for he defines clearly, and not only by his commitment but by his simple presence, in which sphere one is moving. He will be able to contribute helpful responses and clarifications. In fact, it is not simply a matter of words, but of well-defined themes which preoccupy the sick person: the need for forgiveness, love and hope.

The spiritual response to these needs is also found in a history and a tradition, that of salvation. When the 'humanist' and individual approach fails, it is comforting to know that one is not alone and that one can subscribe to a doctrine and an observance which offer a framework for doubt and anguish. This 'work' on oneself, with someone who is available and prepared, strengthened by prayer, allows one to reach a level which goes beyond destructive destiny. Of course, there is no question of imposing a system of belief which is not the patient's own, or of believing that one is called on to profit by the situation to 'lead a soul to God'. It is simply a matter of being available for a spiritual opening-up (Huber 1976; Conrad 1985).

SUPPORT FOR THE RELATIVES

When the disease is terminal, it is necessary to facilitate the preparation for mourning, without shooting ahead to the detriment of what the patient perhaps still expects from life. The members of the family may be too bound up in daily activity or in the denial of essential problems and feelings to allow us to approach them without a certain preparation. A good lead into the subject is to suggest to them supplementary resources to help them with a specific task. This is a possible way of seeing how each person reorganizes his position. In fact, when someone is ill or an invalid, a redistribution of roles is necessary and naturally depends on the style of the family and the degree of interdependence of its members.

Supplementary tasks, the overloading of someone who has no vocation for it, and changes in roles (particularly that of the wife, who suddenly has to deal with the province reserved up till now for the husband) may lead to feelings of usurpation or of disloyalty, or on the other hand of incompetence, or to conflicts of competence. Equalizing tasks and consolidating resources allows them to return to a certain solidarity and to sharing responsibilities, which improves everyone's quality of life (Cantore 1978).

Although the fatal outcome of the illness is often known as much by the patient as by the adult members of the family, this perspective is often not discussed among them. Each player in the drama struggles on his own, often with a fragmented view of the global problem. To achieve a change in the style of communication, suffering and difficulties must be acknowledged by everyone.

Emotional interdependence generally involves a hypersensitivity to the subjects which disturb the other person and which will be instinctively avoided. It is well understood that death is one of the taboo subjects which most threatens the functional equilibrium of a family. If the expression of feelings is banned, the shock wave provoked by the cancer and its consequences cannot be absorbed, and the family will cover up the emotional upheaval which accompanies it. Anguish, sadness, resentment or guilt will then take roundabout routes before dying down, in the form of a demand for extra care, a trivialization of suffering, or a total flight from the situation.

Working with families comprises various levels of assessment. I have already mentioned the style appropriate to the family, its rules, its habits and its way of communicating. There is also, of course, the stage of the life cycle which they have reached, generally according to the age of the children. The approach will be considerably modified according to whether they are small, adolescents or adults. When the unity of the family is threatened, small children react in their own way, and various studies show clearly that the parent in good health very rarely comes to share with them the right amount of information and feeling, without either keeping them out of things or over-burdening them. The great risks for adolescents are of blocking the process of emancipation and of involvement in the too-heavy tasks of parentification. These tasks are perhaps normal, and to a certain extent suitable, but there too it is not very easy to allow them to regain their autonomy without speaking first of the expectation of plans, of duties, and of guilt (Wellisch 1979; Singer 1984; Hoerni 1985).

Case study no. 9

Mme M., 40 years old, had been hospitalized for three weeks with a very aggressive cancer. The attempts made to allow her to return home, while there was still time, were frustrated by reason of multiple pain that could not be relieved. The patient was married and had two children aged 6 and 8. Around her there was much 'technical' activity. During the interviews with the psychiatrist, she came to speak of her anguish, of death, of her guilt in neglecting her role of mother and wife, and above all of her anxiety in entrusting all her tasks to her husband, whom she considered a great baby, incapable of managing on his own.

Relaxation exercises and suitable medication enabled her to deal with her blocks, to diminish her feeling of worthlessness and her disgust for her body, which had led her to refuse visits from her children. Several joint interviews restored the husband's self-esteem and allowed him to clarify his ideas about the children's education. It was agreed that a home help would take over the housework, and that nursing care, medical help, and a hospital bed would be laid on. With this preparation, the patient accepted her return home. Her room would be arranged in the living room on the ground floor, according to the husband's instructions and the authority delegated to him. Mme M. would thus be able, to a certain extent, to regain the central position which she occupied in her family, but by delegating the major role to her husband, who from now on had a definite task to perform. Her anguish was then channelled.

The children became used to the presence of their sick mother, and shared with her their daily concerns. A fortnight later, the patient died at home, without excessive suffering, in the presence of her family and of the treating physician. The children were able to kiss her, to be present at the death, and to touch her body. Their emotional reactions were talked over at length with their father and the doctor, who maintained contact with the children as long as necessary. Six months later, they can speak of their mother with sadness but quite naturally, and they still feel her presence among them. The father still shows that he is up to his tasks.

Families who experience the most difficulty in coping with the situation often have a long history of problems, particularly in relation to existential stages, old griefs, conflicts, or stress. Often they give the impression of having very open conversations, but these may perhaps encourage group unity in the face of adversity, by excluding everything which risks conflict, to the detriment of the feeling and individuality of its members. Our intervention should support cohesion by defining needs and priorities, by finding the means of help and support for each one to open up communication (Matthews Simonton 1984).

It is often forgotten that the disease, its mutilations and its treatments may engender various degrees of fear and loathing. A partner or children will be disconcerted by the changes in behaviour or the deterioration of their loved one and will be hypersensitive to their appearance. Feelings of rage, sadness, or depression about what is happening can be intense. This is an intolerable assault on the ideal picture of the family group. These negative feelings, even if they are addressed more to the situation than to the patient himself, will be extremely difficult to express. Guilt at experiencing them is a further barrier to communication.

Case study no. 10

Mlle S., 68 years old, was suffering from terminal cancer, originally of the breast. Living far from her relatives, she suddenly came into conflict with her doctors, and had herself transferred to the hospital in the town where most of her family lived.

The youngest of a family of four, with a twin brother, she had taken care of her parents until their death. The family knew that she had had a relationship with a married man, but disapproved of it. This friend had died two years earlier, a few months before the appearance of the cancer. The psychiatrist was called to the patient, who had breathing difficulties that were clinically inexplicable. In fact, he understood indirectly that this call came from a sister-in-law who spent her days beside Mlle S. The interview with the patient allowed her to speak of her resentment towards this rather intrusive sister-in-law, and towards her relatives, who gave her no credit for having sacrificed herself for them all. She regretted only seeing one member of the family by marriage. A family reunion was organized with her agreement, reuniting the brothers and sister. An intense feeling of guilt was noticeable, as was the impossibility of getting close to the patient, owing to ancient feuds. The most inhibited turned out to be the twin brother. After the clearing up of certain emotional problems and the manifestation of the proper family way of dealing with situations of mourning, the twin brother decided to pay a visit to his sister. In the presence of the psychiatrist, they were able to speak of their common memories. Both made a reckoning of the qualities and virtues which they saw in each other, the pleasures and the pain which they had shared. The patient received acknowledgement for her devotion and for her sacrifice of certain personal potentialities for the sake of the family as a whole. During the days that followed, she felt subjectively better and was able to receive the other members of the family, one by one. A week later, she died during the night, holding her brother's hand.

We have seen that being ill requires considerable readjustment, the renunciation of certain expectations, which is reinforced by the proximity of death. For mourning to begin, the individual must confront his feelings in relation to the alteration of what he is with regard to himself and others. The sadness which is so important at such times may be minimized or denied, so as to avoid pain. Experiences in the past which have been ill accepted sometimes alter the perception of reality.

As new roles and new demands overload the members of the family, resentment and confusion will easily arise. As appreciated roles have contributed to self-esteem, their inevitable renunciation will lead to feelings of worthlessness and depression. Death brings about fear and aggression, just at a time when these emotions are not very acceptable. This reinforces guilt still more, and the tendency to deny reality, while favouring the idealization of the one who is going to die. The inability to accept contradictory emotions which are bound up with death blocks the process of separation in its course, and anger or resentment are displaced onto other members of the family, onto the medical team, or onto the patient himself (Crisp 1986).

To help the family as well as the patient to face up to reality and to the intense feelings associated with it encourages mourning. Open and fruitful communication introduces the possibility of saying goodbye. This is the culmination of their life in common and the sharing of the last wishes for the future. Sometimes, permission may be given for remarriage.

To say goodbye is to recognize that one has been a good partner or a good son, or to discover that one has really been loved. In the cases where it has not been possible to complete this unfinished business, the survivor tells of how much he is haunted by questions which he would have liked to ask while there was still time. The last words of a dying person always have a great moral force. And so a positive experience of saying goodbye, of taking care and of forgiveness has an extraordinary validity and is full of richness for the survivors. After the death and after the funeral, the survivors remain with a past which has ceased to be and a present where the pain of loss and mourning are alive. At this time the widower or widow must be able to maintain relationships with the health-care team.

Death – the final event – provokes an intense reaction. Once more, feelings of sadness must be expressed. To recognize the fears of being alone or feeling inadequate for the work of reintegration may be useful. It is possible that a survivor may feel ill at ease with the hospital system, for he has reproaches to express; he needs to go over the story to determine where mistakes were made. Feelings of guilt and aggression will interfere with grief. Functional symptoms may arise, imitating those of the deceased by identification. One must try to link these symptoms with the loss of the loved one and help the survivor to understand the evolution of such symptomatology, without falling into the vicious circle of the quest for an organic illness. In order to discourage excessive identification or fusion with the image of the deceased, the process of individuation must be reinforced, by valuing the achievements and personal worth of the survivor.

Case study no. 11

Mlle B., aged 30, lived in a state of insurmountable grief for three years, following the death of her boyfriend, caused by a lymphoma. She had supported him in his illness for several years, identifying completely with him. She was valued by the whole oncological medical team as the ideal companion, devoted and efficient. Shortly after the death, she gave up work and started consulting several doctors for multiple functional disorders; she finally consulted psychiatrists, all of whom abandoned the attempt to treat her because of her 'lack of motivation'. Her stubborn streak made her the doctors' *bête noire*. Desperate, she ended by making contact with the psychiatrist in the department where her friend had died. She considered this doctor as a member of her new 'oncological' family, and therefore likely to understand her. To sum up, many sessions of psychotherapy resulted in the protection and validation of her grief as her most precious possession, which could only be mentioned with her consent, and this greatly relaxed the atmosphere. She appeared more receptive, progressively abandoning her position of all-powerful and hostile withdrawal. It was only after several months that she was finally able to speak of herself and of her links with her own family. It was clear that no process of individuation had been started, and that she had left her relatives abruptly to live with her boyfriend. She had nevertheless felt that she should continue doing many jobs for her family, to the detriment of her own interests. Incapable of expressing her own feelings, she projected everything onto others, above all transferring responsibility for her present unhappiness on to her parents. It was only after having given up the hope that her parents would change that she interrupted a new university course and began to portray her isolation and her tragedy.

Having regained a certain personal equilibrium, little by little she emerged from her immense sadness and rediscovered the meaning of her existence. During the later sessions she appeared much more animated and autonomous and was able to speak of her desire for pregnancy, which was always refused by her boyfriend, and of all the bitterness and nostalgia which she felt towards him for having abandoned her.

Grief has been at the centre of this last chapter. It is perhaps strange to end with such a theme, but it seems to me to be at the core of the resources available to deal with the emotions of every individual and of every family. When it is a question of cancer, people – relatives or the sick themselves – in fact fear irreparable loss more than death, and they are confronted by a sort of balance-sheet of their life.

The French word *deuil* represents several phenomena that the English language has been able to differentiate in terms that are adapted to quite distinct processes: the loss of a loved one (*bereavement*) and the feeling of deep sadness and despair that accompanies it (*grief*), which both form part of a wider whole, evolving for the entire length of our existence, which is the capacity to lament losses, disappointments, and changes that have been overcome (no longer to grieve, but to *mourn*). *Mourning* begins at the early stage of life and reaches its maturity after adolescence, when the psychic equipment is developed.

These definitions are important for, at the moment of reaching the illness or the death of one of its members (whether it has taken place or is anticipated), the family will react not only according to the experience or the dynamic of the moment, but also according to past experience. These are the heritage and loyalties which are transmitted in a more or less unconscious way through several generations and which correspond to the way in which the experiences of breakup and change have been overcome over time. The heritage of mourning includes not only the loss of loved ones but also uprootings, nostalgia for one's origins, and all the abstractions built into moral beings (patrimony, liberty, ideals, and so on).

And so death, as the ultimate loss, reactivates the universal pain of separation. Often, the development or abatement of this pain has taken time and energy, or even produced the appearance of a scarcely healed catastrophe, to the point sometimes that the fear of reliving a similar experience is a sufficiently powerful motive to bring about among some people avoidance or denial of everything which distances or removes even symbolically. One may take, as examples, the passing of time and the stages of growing old, the individuation and then the emancipation of children, but quite obviously also an illness such as cancer. Mourning that was not carried out in a previous generation may thus be at the source of the most rigid resistances of a family as regards what is or is not acceptable. Before speaking to someone about 'mourning', it therefore seems crucial to determine in which personal and family history death is, or will be, inscribed.

Very often, mourning is a normal process, complex, active, which occurs like any other existential event. It usually develops on its own and within a limited period (six months to a year), even if it is almost always accompanied by a change in one's view of the world, with above all an exacerbation of the loss of one's own feeling of invulnerability. To grieve is to be able to feel unhappy, which includes moral distress, depression, uncontrollable weeping, the feeling of isolation, a certain irritability and intense anguish. After a certain period, the spontaneous grief work will aim at removing some of the emotional attachment that one bears towards the one who is no longer, so as to facilitate investment in new relationships and activities. But this is not always possible, for a certain number of risk factors may play a blocking role, to the extent that they introduce other priorities and get in the way of the freedom to give rein to depression and despondency:

- the needs and demands of children and dependent members of the family (for example, a mother who suddenly has to take on the responsibilities of the father);
- problems of finance and housing;
- the lack of a near relation or of adequate support at difficult times;
- a sociocultural system that inhibits the expression of feelings;
- repeated losses of relationships;
- family or marital conflicts, and resulting disputes which were not resolved at the time of death;
- pre-existing psychiatric or psychological problems.

If one meets the family only after the death of a relative, because of pathological or masked grief manifesting in psychiatric or somatic symptomatology, one must attempt a recentring by recalling the event, remembering life with the deceased, the feelings which sustained him and the place that everyone occupied at that time. In this way one can gain a picture of the way in which structures and communication have been reorganized, with what kind of allocation of roles. Setbacks at school or truancy in an adolescent, for example, may be a way of supporting a depressive mother after the death of her husband, enabling the student to stay at home to prevent the realization of the suffering caused by the empty space.

To work through mourning that has been blocked, it is necessary to begin everything from the beginning in a sort of 'regriefing', that is, a reactivation of the grief which allows emotions to be revitalized, so as to prevent the redistribution of family roles being a way of over-occupying the place of the deceased, with all the ambiguity and pathological potential that this represents. It is a matter of accepting the reality of the loss, and of achieving adaptation to an environment where there is a gap, without wishing to fill it at all costs. It is only in this way that families and individuals can evolve and regain the feeling of controlling life, which can then continue without the one who is missing.

Bibliography

Abse, D. (1964) 'Investigative psychotherapy and cancer', in D.M. Kissen and L.L. LeShan (eds) *Psychosomatic aspects of neoplastic disease*, London: Pitman.

Abse, D.W., Wilkins, M.M, Buxton, W.D., *et al.* (1973) 'Personality and behavioral characteristics of lung cancer patients', *Journal of Psychosomatic Research* 18: 101–9.

Ader, R. (1975) 'Behaviorally conditioned immunosuppression', *Psychosomatic Medicine* 37: 333–40.

Ahrens, S. (1979) 'Interaktionsmuster der ambulanten Arzt. Patient-Beziehung in der Allgemeinpraxis', in J.F. Siegrist and A. Hendel-Kramer (eds) *Wege zum Arzt*, Munich: Urban & Schwarzenberg, 83–112.

Alexander, F.M. (1932) *The use of the self* (new edition 1985), London: Gollancz.

Alexander, G. (1971) *L'eutonie*, Paris: Editions du Scarabée.

Allen, A. (1979) 'Psychiatry and the oncology unit', *The Psychiatric Journal of the University of Ottawa* IV: 213–6.

Alvin, J. (1975) *Music Therapy*, London: Hutchinson.

American College of Physicians (1983) 'Drug therapy for severe chronic pain in terminal illness', *Annals of Internal Medicine* 99: 870–3.

American Medical Association, Department of Drugs (1980) 'General analgesics', in *AMA Drug Evaluations*, 4th edition, New York: Wiley, 55–85.

Andersen, B.L. and Hacker, N.F. 1983) 'Treatment for gynecologic cancer: a review of effects on female sexuality', *Health Psychology* 2: 203–21.

Arkko, P.J., Arkko, B.L., Kari-Koskinen, O., *et al.* (1980) 'A survey of unproven cancer remedies and their uses in an outpatient clinic for cancer therapy in Finland', *Social Science & Medicine* 14A: 511–14.

Asken, M.J. (1975) 'Psychoemotional aspects of mastectomy: a review of recent literature', *American Journal of Psychiatry* 132: 56.

Bahnson, C.B. (1969) 'Psychophysiological complementarity in malignancies: past work and future vistas', *New York Academy of Sciences. Annals* 164: 319–34.

—— (1975) 'Psychologic and emotional issues in cancer: the psychotherapeutic care of the cancer patient', *Seminars in Oncology* 2: 293–308.

—— (1976) 'Emotional and personality characteristics of cancer patients', in A.I. Sutnick and P.F. Engstrom (eds) *Oncology medicine*, Baltimore: University Park Press.

—— (1980) 'Stress and cancer: the state of the art', *Psychosomatics* 21: 975.

Bahnson, C.B. and Bahnson, M.B. (1964) 'Denial and repression of primitive impulses and of disturbing emotions in patients with malignant neoplasms', in D.M. Kissen and L.L. LeShan (eds) *Psychosomatic aspects of neoplastic disease*, London: Pitman.

—— (1966) 'Role of the ego defenses: denial and repression in the etiology of malignant neoplasm', *New York Academy of Sciences. Annals* 125: 827–45.

Balint, M. and Balint, E. (1961) *Psychotherapeutic techniques in medicine*, London: Tavistock.

Baltrusch, H.J.F. (1956) 'Persönlichkeitsstruktur und Erkrankung. Die Rolle emotionaler Faktoren im Krankheitsgeschehen', *Medizinische Klinik* 34: 69–76.

—— (1975) 'Ergebnisse klinisch-psychosomatischer Krebsforschung', *Psychosomatische Medizin* 5: 175–208.

Baltrusch, H.J.F. and Waltz, M. (1985) 'Cancer from a biobehavioral and social epidemiological perspective', *Social Science & Medicine* 20: 789–94.

Bammer, K. (1981) *Krebs und Psychosomatik*, Stuttgart: Kohlhammer.

Bannerman, R.H., Burton, J., and Wen-Chieh, C. (1983) *Traditional medicine and health care coverage*, Geneva: World Health Organization.

Barlow, W. (1973) *The Alexander principle*, London: Gollancz.

Barrett Noone, R., Frazier, T.G., Hayward, C.Z., *et al.* (1982) 'Patient acceptance of immediate reconstruction following mastectomy', *Plastic and Reconstructive Surgery* 69: 632.

Barsky, A.J. and Brown, H.N. (1982) 'Psychiatric teaching and consultation in a primary care clinic', *Psychosomatics* 23: 908–21.

Bartuska, D.G. (1975) 'Humoral manifestations of neoplasms', *Seminars in Oncology* 2: 405–9.

Benoliel, J.Q. (1985) 'Loss and terminal illness', *Nursing Clinics of North America* 20: 439–48.

Benson, H. (1975) *The relaxation response*, New York: Morrow.

Benson, H., Rosner, B.E., Marzetta, B.R., and Klemchuck, H.M. (1974) 'Decreased blood pressure in pharmacologically treated hypertensive patients who regularly elicited the relaxation response', *Lancet* (i): 289–91.

Bernstein, I.L., Wallace, M.J., Bernstein, I.D., *et al.* (1979) 'Learned food aversions as a consequence of cancer treatment', in J. van Eys, M.S. Seelig, and B.L. Nichols (eds) *Nutrition and Cancer*, New York: SP Medical & Scientific Books, 159–64.

Bertakis, K.D. (1977) 'The communication of information from physician to patient', *Journal of Family Practice* 5: 217–22.

Bertalanffy, L. von (1964) 'The mind-body problem: a new view', *Psychosomatic Medicine* 26: 29–45.

Bishop, B. (1985) *A time to heal*, London: Severn House.

Blackie, M. (1986) *Classical homeopathy*, Beaconsfield: Beaconsfield Publishers.

Bloom, J.R. (1982) 'Social support, accommodation to stress and adjustment to breast cancer', *Social Science & Medicine* 16: 1329–38.

Boltanski, L. (1971) 'Les usages sociaux du corps', *Annales – Economies, Sociétiés, Civilisations* 1: 205–33.

Bonhoeffer, K. (1974) 'Exogenous psychoses', in S.R. Hirsch and I.M. Shepard (eds) *Themes and variations in European psychiatry*, Bristol: J. Wright & Sons, 47–52.

Bonica, J.J. (1979) 'Importance of the problem', in J.J. Bonica, V. Ventafridda, R.B. Fink, *et al.* (eds) *Advances in pain research and therapy*, vol. 2, New York: Raven Press, 1–12.

Booth, G. (1969) 'General and organ-specific object relationships in cancer', *New York Academy of Sciences. Annals* 164: 568–74.

Boszormenyi-Nagy, I. and Spark, G.M. (1973) *Invisible loyalties*, New York: Harper & Row.

Boudon, P. (1979) 'La représentation du corps dans la pensée et la médecine chinoise', *Anthropologica* 21: 73–120.

Bovbjerg, D. (1989) 'Psychoneuroimmunology and cancer', in J.C. Holland and J.H. Rowland (eds) *Handbook of psychooncology: psychological care of the patient with cancer*, New York: Oxford University Press, 727–34.

Bransfield, D.D. (1982–3) 'Breast cancer and sexual functioning: a review of the literature and implications for future research', *International Journal of Psychiatry in Medicine* 12 (3): 197–211.

Bristor, M.W. (1984) 'Birth of a handicapped child: a wholistic model for grieving', *Family Relations* 33: 30-1.

Broad, W.J. (1978) 'New laetrile study leaves cancer institute in the pits', *Science* 202: 33–6.

Brohn, P. (1986) *Gentle Giants*, London: Century.

Bronner-Huszar, J. (1971) 'The psychological aspects of cancer in man', *Psychosomatics* 12: 133–8.

Brown, H.J. and Paraskevas, F. (1982) 'Cancer and depression. Cancer presenting with depressive illness: an autoimmune disease', *British Journal of Psychiatry* 141: 227–32.

Buber, M. (1937) *I and Thou*, Edinburgh: T. & T. Clark.

Burish, T.G. and Bradley, L.A. (1983) *Coping with chronic disease*, New York: Academic Press.

Burish, T.G. and Lyles, J.N. (1979) 'Effectiveness of relaxation training in reducing the aversiveness of chemotherapy in the treatment of cancer', *Behavior Therapy & Experimental Psychiatry* 10: 357–61.

Cadwell, D. (1986) 'Healing', *Health Visitor* 59: 347.

Cameron, E. and Pauling, L. (1979) *Cancer and vitamin C*, New York: Warner.

Cantore, R.C. (1978) *And a time to live: toward emotional well-being during the crisis of cancer*, New York: Harper & Row.

Capone, M.A., Goods, R.S., Westie, K.S., *et al.* (1980) 'Psychosocial rehabilitation of gynecologic oncology patients', *Archives of Physical Medicine and Rehabilitation* 61: 128–32.

Carey, R. (1974) 'Emotional adjustment in terminal patients; a quantitative approach', *Journal of Counseling Psychology* 21: 433–9.

Carkhuff, R.R. (1969) *Helping and human relations: a primer for lay and professional helpers*, vols I and II, New York: Holt, Rinehart & Winston.

Certeau, M. de (1975) 'Ecrire l'innommable', in 'Lieux et objets de la mort', *Traverses* 1: 9–16.

Chapman, C. (1979) 'Psychologic and behavioral aspects of pain', in J.J. Bonica, V. Ventafridda, R.B. Fink, *et al.* (eds) *Advances in pain research and therapy*, vol. 2, New York: Raven Press, 45–56.

Chapman, R.M., Sutcliffe, S.B., and Malpas, J.S. (1981) 'Male gonadal dysfunction in Hodgkin's disease', *J A M A: The Journal of the American Medical Association* 245: 1323–8.

Chardot, C. (1984) 'De la formation psychologique du médecin spécialiste en cancérologie', *Psychologie Médicale* 16: 2195–6.

Chopra, D. (1989) *Quantum healing*, New York: Bantam.

Christensen, S. and Harding, M. (1985) 'Integration theories of crisis intervention into hospice home care teaching', *Nursing Clinics of North America* 20: 449–55.

Cleeland, C.S. (1984) 'The impact of pain on patients with cancer', *Cancer* 53: 2635–41.

Clover, A. (1992) 'Complementary cancer care', *British Homeopathic Journal* 81 (4): 176–82.

Cobb, S. and Erbe, C. (1978) 'Social support for the cancer patient', *Forum on Medicine* 1: 24–9.

Cobliner, W.G. (1977) 'Psychological factors in gynecological or breast malignancies', *Hospital Physician*: 38–40.

Connell, C. (1992) 'Art therapy as part of a palliative care programme', *Palliative Medicine* 6: 18–24.

Conrad, N.L. (1985) 'Spiritual support for the dying', *Nursing Clinics of North America* 20: 415–26.

Contrada, R.J., Leventhal, H., and O'Leary, A. (1990) 'Personality and health', in L.A. Pervin (ed.) *Handbook of personality: theory and research*, New York: Guilford, 638–69.

Cooter, R. (ed.) (1988) *Studies in the history of alternative medicine*, Basingstoke: Macmillan.

Cosh, J. and Sikora, K. (1989) 'Conventional and complementary treatments for cancer: time to join forces', *British Medical Journal* 298: 1200–1.

Craig, T.L. and Abeloff, M.D. (1974) 'Psychiatric symptomatology among hospitalized cancer patients', *American Journal of Pyschiatry* 141: 1323–7.

Crisp, A.H. (1986) 'Le processus du deuil', *Hexagone 'Roche'* 14: 12–17.

Dean, C., Chetty, U., and Forrest, A.P.M. (1983) 'Effects of immediate breast reconstruction on psychosocial morbidity after mastectomy', *Lancet* (i): 459–62.

Degenaar, J.J. (1979) 'Some philosophical considerations on pain', *Pain* 7: 281–304.

Derogatis, L.R. (1982) 'Psychopharmacologic applications to cancer', *Cancer* 50: 1962–7.

Derogatis, L.R., Abeloff, M.D., and Melisaratos, N. (1979a) 'Psychological coping mechanisms and survival time in metastatic breast cancer',

J A M A: The Journal of the American Medical Association 242: 1504–8.

Derogatis, L.R., Feldstein, M., Morrow, G., *et al.* (1979b) 'A survey of psychotropic drug prescriptions in an oncology population', *Cancer* 44: 1919–29.

Derogatis, L.R. and Kourlesis, S.M. (1981a) 'An approach to evaluation of sexual problems in the cancer patient', *Ca – A Cancer Journal for Clinicians* 31: 46–50.

Derogatis, L.R., Meyer, J.K., and King, K.M. (1981b) 'Psychopathology in individuals with sexual dysfunction', *American Journal of Psychiatry* 138: 757–63.

Derogatis, L.R., Morrow, G.R., Fetting, J., *et al.* (1983) 'The prevalence of psychiatric disorders among cancer patients', *J A M A: The Journal of the American Medical Association* 249: 751–7.

DeWys, W.D. (1979) 'Anorexia as a general effect of cancer', *Cancer* 43: 2013–19.

Doll, R. and Peto, R. (1981) *The causes of cancer*, New York: Oxford University Press.

Dufey, D.L., Hamerman, D., and Cohen, M.A. (1980) 'Communication skills of house officers', *Annals of Internal Medicine* 93: 354–7.

Dundee, J. (1988) 'Acupuncture/acupressure as an antiemetic: studies of its use in postoperative vomiting, cancer chemotherapy and sickness of early pregnancy', *Complementary Medical Research* 3: 1, 2–14.

Dutz, W., Kohout, E., Rossipal, E., *et al.* (1976) 'Infantile stress, immune modulation and disease patterns', *Pathology Annual* 11: 415–54.

Eich, E., Reeves, J.L., Jaeger, B., *et al.* (1985) 'Memory of pain: relation between past and present pain intensity', *Pain* 23: 375–9.

Eisenberg, D.M., Kessler, R.C., Foster, C. *et al.* (1993) 'Unconventional medicine in the United States', *New England Journal of Medicine* 328 (4): 246–52.

Eisendrath, S.J. (1981) 'Psychiatric liaison support groups for general hospital staffs', *Psychosomatics* 22: 685–94.

Eliade, M. (1978) *Le chamanisme*, Paris: Payothèque.

Endicott, J. (1984) 'Measurement of depression in patients with cancer', *Cancer* 53: 2243–8.

Engel, G.L. (1977) 'The need for a new medical model: a challenge for biomedicine', *Science* 196: 129–36.

Engel, G.L. and Romano, J. (1959) 'Delirium: a syndrome of cerebral insufficiency', *Journal of Chronic Diseases* 9: 260–77.

Epstein, S. (1976) 'Anxiety, arousal, and the self-concept', in I.G. Sarason and C.D. Spielberger (eds) *Stress and anxiety*, vol. 3, Washington, D.C.: Hemisphere.

Euster, S.E. (1979) 'Rehabilitation after mastectomy: the group process', *Social Work in Health Care* 4: 251–63.

Evans, E. (1926) *A psychological study of cancer*, New York: Dodd, Mead & Co.

Fain, M. (1966) 'Régression et psychosomatique', *Revue Française de Psychanalyse* 30: 451–6.

Falek, A. and Britton, S. (1974) 'Phases in coping: the hypothesis and its implications', *Social Biology* 21: 1–7.

Fallowfield, L. (1990) *The quality of life: the missing measurement in health care*, London: Souvenir.

Fankhauser, H. (1986) 'Rôle du neurochirurgien dans la consultation multidisciplinaire de la douleur chronique', *Revue Médicale de la Suisse Romande* 106: 1047–54.

Farberow, N.L., Shneidman, E.S., and Leonard, C.V. (1964) 'Suicide among general medical and surgical hospital patients with malignant neoplasms', *The New Physician* 38–44.

Feldenkrais, M. (1972) *Awareness through movement: health exercises for personal growth*, New York: Harper & Row.

Feldman, F.L. (1978) 'Work and cancer health histories', American Cancer Society, California Division, Oakland.

Ferlic, M., Goldman, A., and Kennedy, B.J. (1979) 'Group counselling in adult patients with advanced cancer', *Cancer* 43: 760–6.

Fetting, J.H., Grochow, L.B., Folstein, J.F., *et al.* (1982) 'The course of nausea and vomiting after high-dose Cyclophosphamide', *Cancer Treatment Reports* 66: 1487–93.

Fetting, J.H., Wilcox, P.M., Iwata, B.A., *et al.* (1983) 'Anticipatory nausea and vomiting in an ambulatory oncology population', *Cancer Treatment Reports* 67: 1090–8.

Fisher, S. (1967) 'Motivation for patients' delay', *Archives of General Psychiatry* 16: 676–8.

Fitts, W.T., Jr and Ravdin, I.S. (1953) 'What Philadelphia physicians tell patients with cancer', *J A M A: The Journal of the American Medical Association* 153: 901–4.

Foley, K.M. (1982) 'The practical use of narcotic analgesics', *Medical Clinics of North America* 66: 1091–104.

—— (1985) 'The treatment of cancer pain', *New England Journal of Medicine* 313 (2): 84–95.

Folkman, S., Schaefer, C., and Lazarus, R.S. (1979) 'Cognitive processes as mediators of stress and coping', in V. Hamilton and D.M. Warburton (eds) *Human stress and cognition: an information processing approach*, London: Wiley.

Folstein, M.F., Fetting, J.H., Lobo, A., *et al.* (1984) 'Cognitive assessment of cancer patients', *Cancer* 53: 2250–5.

Forester, B., Kornfeld, D.S., and Fleiss, J.L. (1985) 'Psychotherapy during radiotherapy: effects on emotional and physical distress', *American Journal of Psychiatry* 142: 22–7.

Fortini, K. and Wyss, F. (1985) 'Que penser du deuil chez la personne âgée?', *Médecine & Hygiène* 43: 3529–33.

Fox, B.H. (1978) 'Premorbid psychological factors as related to cancer incidence', *Journal of Behavioral Medicine* 1: 45–65.

Frankl, V.E. (1962) *Man's search for meaning*, Boston: Beacon Press.

Freidenbergs, I., Gordon, W., Hibbard, M., *et al.* (1981–2) 'Psychosocial aspects of living with cancer: a review of the literature', *International Journal of Psychiatry in Medicine* 11: 303–29.

Friedman, H.S. (1970) 'Physician management of dying patients: an exploration', *Psychiatric Medicine* 1: 295–305.

Fulder, S. (1988) *The handbook of complementary medicine*, Oxford: Oxford University Press.

158 An introduction to psycho-oncology

Futz, J.M. and Senay, E.C. (1975) 'Guidelines for management of hospitalized narcotic addicts', *Annals of Internal Medicine* 82: 815–8.

Gendron, D. (1701) *Inquiries into the nature, knowledge and cure of cancer*, London.

Georgiades, G.S., Riefkohl, R., Cox, E., *et al.* (1985) 'Long-term clinical outcome of immediate reconstruction after mastectomy', *Plastic and Reconstructive Surgery* 76: 415.

Gerson, M. (1990) *A cancer therapy: results of fifty cases*, ed. G. Hildenbrand, New York: Gerson Institute.

Goland, N. (1981) *Passage through transitions*, New York: Free Press.

Goldberg, R. and Cullen, L.O. (1985) 'Factors important to psychosocial adjustment to cancer: a review of the evidence', *Social Science & Medicine* 20: 803–7.

Goldberg, R. and Tull, R.M. (1983) *The psychosocial dimensions of cancer*, New York: Free Press.

Golden, S. (1975) 'Cancer chemotherapy and management of patient problems', *Nursing Forum* 12: 279–303.

Gordon, W., Freidenbergs, I., Diller, L., *et al.* (1980) 'Efficacy of psychosocial intervention with cancer patients', *Journal of Consulting and Clinical Psychology* 48: 743–59.

Gorzynski, J.G. and Holland, J.C. (1979) 'Psychological aspects of testicular cancer', *Seminars in Oncology* 6: 125–9.

Gottlieb, B.H. (1981) 'Preventive interventions involving social networks and social support', in B.H. Gottlieb (ed.) *Social networks and social support*, Beverly Hills: Sage, 201–32.

Gottschalk, L.A. (1984) 'Measurement of mood and affect in cancer patients', *Cancer* 53: 2236–41.

Greenberg, R.P. and Dattore, P.J. (1981) 'The relationship between dependency and the development of cancer', *Psychosomatic Medicine* 43: 35–43.

Greenblatt, D.J., Shader, R.I., and Koch-Weser, J. (1975) 'Psychotropic drug use in the Boston area', *Archives of General Psychiatry* 32: 518–21.

Greene, W.A. (1966) 'The psychosocial setting of the development of leukemia and lymphoma', *New York Academy of Sciences. Annals.* 125: 794–801.

Greer, S. (1984) 'The psychological dimension in cancer treatment', *Social Science & Medicine* 18: 345–9.

Greer, S., Moorey, S., Baruch, J.D.R., *et al.* (1992) 'Adjuvant psychological therapy for patients with cancer: a prospective randomised trial', *British Medical Journal* 304: 675–80.

Greer, S. and Morris, T. (1975) 'Psychological attributes of women who develop breast cancer: a controlled study', *Journal of Psychosomatic Research* 19: 147–53.

Greer, S., Morris, T., and Pettingale, K.W. (1979) 'Psychological response to breast cancer: effect on outcome', *Lancet* (ii): 785–7.

Greer, S. and Watson, M. (1985) 'Towards a psychobiological model of cancer: psychological considerations', *Social Science & Medicine* 20: 773–7.

Guck, T.P., Skultety, M., Meilman, P.W., *et al.* (1985) 'Multidisciplinary

Pain Center follow-up study: evaluation with a no-treatment control group', *Pain* 21: 295–306.

Guex, P. (1982) 'Le dialogue jusqu'à la mort: un accompagnement par la prescription de soi-même', *Médecine & Hygiène* 40: 2261–2.

—— (1983) 'Pourquoi les patients cancéreux ont-ils recours aux médecines parallèles? – Une perspective psychologique', *Schweizerische Rundschau für Medizin Praxis* 72: 49–52.

—— (1984) 'Les relations médecins-guérisseurs dans une consultation de cancérologie: lutte ou intégration fantasmatique?', *Psychologie Médicale* 16: 1159–60.

—— (1986a) 'Approche psychologique du problème des reconstructions mammaires', *Swiss Review for Medicine and Medical Technique* 6a: 26–7.

—— (1986b) 'Douleur chronique et relation médecin–malade (La fonction du symptôme douleur)', *Revue Médicale de la Suisse Romande* 106: 1031–4.

—— (1986c) 'Le cancéreux et la famille', *Médecine & Hygiène*, suppl. to no. 1670: 10–12.

Guex, P., Carron, R., Barrelet, L., et al. (1983) 'Guérison subjective du cancer et communication', Psychologie Médicale 15: 1557–60.

Guex, P. and Barrelet, L. (1984) 'Rôle du consultant psychiatre dans la formation de l'équipe soignante et la prise en charge des patients d'une consultation de cancérologie', *Psychologie Médicale* 16: 2261–2.

Guex, P. and MacDonald, S. (1984) 'Le rôle d'un groupe de relaxation-eutonie dans l'amélioration de la qualité de vie de patients cancéreux', *Médecine & Hygiène* 42: 2898–902.

Guy, R. (1759) *Essay on squirrhous tumours and cancer*, London: W. Owen.

Hackett, T.P. and Cassem, N.H. (1974) 'Development of a quantitative rating scale to assess denials', *Journal of Psychosomatic Research* 18: 93–100.

Hackett, T.P., Cassem, N.H., and Raker, J.W. (1973) 'Patient delay in cancer', *New England Journal of Medicine* 289: 14–20.

Haes, J.C.J.M. de, and Knippenberg, F.C.E. van (1985) 'The quality of life of cancer patients: a review of the literature', *Social Science & Medicine* 20: 809–17.

Haes, J.C.J.M. de, Knippenberg, F.C.E. van, and Neijt, J.P. (1990) 'Measuring psychological and physical distress in cancer patients: structure and application of the Rotterdam Symptom Checklist', *British Journal of Cancer* 62: 1034–8.

Hall, N.M. (1991) *Reflexology – a way to better health*, Bath: Gateway.

Halman, M. and Suttinger, J. (1978) 'Family-centered care of cancer patients', *Nursing* 78: 42–3.

Hahnemann, S. (1842) *Organon of medicine*, trans. J. Künzli, A. Navdé, and P. Pendleton (1983), London: Gollancz.

Harwood, A. (1971) 'The hot-cold theory of disease. Implications for treatment of Puerto Rican patients', *J A M A: The Journal of the American Medical Association* 216: 1153–8.

Helson, H. and Bevan, W. (1967) *Contemporary approaches to psychology*, New York: Van Nostrand.

Henderson, J.G. (1966) 'Denial and repression as factors in the delay of patients with cancer presenting themselves to the physicians', *New York Academy of Sciences. Annals* 125: 856–64.

Herberman, R.B. (1982) 'Possible effects of central nervous system on natural killer (NK) cell activity', in S.M. Levy (ed.) *Biological mediators of behavior and disease: neoplasia*, New York: Elsevier Biomedical.

Hinkle, L.E., Christenson, W.N., Kane, F.D., *et al.* (1958) 'An investigation of the relation between life experience, personality characteristics and general susceptibility to illness', *Psychosomatic Medicine* 20: 278–95.

Hochberg, F.H. and Linggood, R. (1979) 'Quality and duration of survival in glioblastoma multiforme', *J A M A: The Journal of the American Medical Association* 241: 1016–18.

Hoerni, B. (1985) *Paroles et silences du médecin*, Paris: Flammarion.

Holland, J.C. (1977) 'Psychological aspects of oncology', *Medical Clinics of North America* 61: 737–48.

—— (1981) 'Why patients seek unproven cancer remedies: a psychological perspective', *Clinical Bulletin* 2: 55–8.

Holland, J.C. and Mastrovito, R. (1980) 'Psychologic adaptation to breast cancer', *Cancer* 46: 1045–52.

Holm, L.-E., Nordevang, E., Halmar, M.-L., *et al.* (1993) 'Treatment failure and dietary habits in women with breast cancer', *Journal of the National Cancer Institute* 85: 32–6.

House, J.S., Robbins, C., and Metzner, H.L. (1982) 'The association of social relationships and activities with mortality: prospective evidence from the Tecumseh Community Health Survey', *American Journal of Epidemiology* 116: 123–40.

Huber, R. (1976) 'L'approche des mourants', *Bulletin du Centre Protestant d'Etudes* 1–2: 5–20.

Ingle, R.J., Burish, T.G., and Wallston, K.A. (1984) 'Conditionability of cancer chemotherapy patients', *Oncology Nursing Forum* 11: 97–102.

Irwin, M.R., Daniels, M., Risch, S.C., *et al.* (1988) 'Plasma cortisol and natural killer cell activity among bereaved women', *Biological Psychiatry* 24: 173–8.

Iyengar, B.K.S. (1988) *The tree of Yoga*, Oxford: Fine Line.

Jamison, K.R., Wellisch, D.K., and Pasnau, R.O. (1978) 'Psychosocial aspects of mastectomy. I: The woman's perspective', *American Journal of Psychiatry* 135: 432–6.

Jansen, M.A. and Muenz, L.R. (1984) 'A retrospective study of personality variables associated with fibrocystic disease and breast cancer', *Journal of Psychosomatic Research* 28: 35–42.

Jones, F.P. (1976) *Body awareness in action: a study of the Alexander technique*, New York: Schocken Books.

Katz, E.R., Kellerman, J., and Siegel, S.E. (1980) 'Behavioral distress in children with cancer undergoing medical procedures: developmental considerations', *Journal of Consulting and Clinical Psychology* 48: 356–65.

Kerr, T.A., Shapira, K., and Roth, M. (1969) 'The relationship between premature death and affective disorders', *British Journal of Psychiatry* 115: 1277–82.

Khwaja, T.A., Dias, C.B., and Pentecost, S. (1986) 'Recent studies on the anticancer activities of mistletoe (*Viscum album*) and its alkaloids', *Oncology* 43: 42–50.

Kissen, D.M. (1963) 'Personality characteristics in males conducive to lung cancer', *British Journal of Medical Psychology* 36: 27–36.

Klagsbrun, S.C. (1970) 'Cancer, emotions and nurses', *American Journal of Psychiatry* 126: 1237–44.

Kleijnen, J., Knipschild, P., and Riet, G. ter (1991) 'Clinical trials of homoeopathy', *British Medical Journal* 302: 316–23.

Kneier, A.W. and Temoshok, L. (1984) 'Repressive coping reactions in patients with malignant melanoma as compared to cardiovascular disease patients', *Journal of Psychosomatic Research* 28: 145–55.

Kocher, R. (1982) 'Psychopharmacologie et douleur du cancer', *Médecine & Hygiène* 40: 19–23.

Koren, M.J. (1986) 'Home-care – Who cares?', *New England Journal of Medicine* 314: 917–20.

Krant, J.J., Beiser, M. and Adler, G. (1976) 'The role of a hospital-based psychosocial unit in terminal cancer illness and bereavement', *Journal of Chronic Diseases* 29: 115–27.

Krant, M.J. (1981) 'Psychosocial impact of gynecologic cancer', *Cancer* 48: 608–12.

Kübler-Ross, E. (1969) *On death and dying*, New York: Macmillan.

—— (1970) 'Psychotherapy for the dying patient', *Current Psychiatric Therapies* 10: 110–17.

—— (1978) *To live until we say good-bye*, Englewood Cliffs, N.J.: Prentice-Hall, Inc.

Lanski, S.B., List, M.A., and Ritter-Sterr, C. (1986) 'Psychosocial consequences of cure', *Cancer* 58: 529–33.

Lazarus, R.S. and Launier, R. (1978) 'Stress-related transactions between person and environment', in L.A. Pervin and M. Lewis (eds) *Perspectives in interactional psychology*, New York: Plenum Press.

Lechner, P. and Kronberger, I. (1990) 'Erfahrungen mit dem Einsatz der Diät-Therapie in der chirurgischen Onkologie', *Aktuelle Ernährungsmedizin* 15: 2, 51–96.

Lee, E.C. and Maguire, G.P. (1975) 'Emotional distress in patients attending a breast clinic', *British Journal of Surgery* 62: 162.

Lee, T., Pappius, E.M., and Goldman, L. (1983) 'Impact of inter-physician communication on the effectiveness of medical consultations', *American Journal of Medicine* 74: 106–12.

Legmen, J.F., DeLisa, J.H., Warren, C.G., *et al.* (1978) 'Cancer rehabilitation: assessment of need, development, and evaluations of a model of care', *Archives of Physical Medicine and Rehabilitation* 59: 410–19.

Leibel, S.A., Pino, Y., Torres, J.L., *et al.* (1980) 'Improved quality of life following radical radiation therapy for early stage carcinoma of prostate', *Urologic Clinics of North America* 7: 593–604.

Leone, L.A. (1982) 'The concept of hospice', *Ca – A Cancer Journal for Clinicians* 32: 141–3.

LeShan, L. L. (1956) 'Some recurrent life history patterns observed in patients with malignant disease', *Journal of Nervous and Mental Disease* 124: 460–5.

—— (1963) 'Untersuchungen zur Persönlichkeit der Krebskranken', *Zeitschrift für Psychosomatische Medizin und Psychoanalyse* 9: 246–53.
—— (1966) 'An emotional life-history pattern associated with neoplastic disease', *New York Academy of Sciences. Annals.* 125: 780–93.
LeShan, L.L. and Gassmann, M.L. (1958) 'Some observations on psychotherapy with patients suffering from neoplastic disease', *American Journal of Psychotherapy* XII: 723–34.
LeShan, L.L. and Worthington, R.E. (1956) 'Personality as a factor in the pathogenesis of cancer', *British Journal of Medical Psychology* 29: 307–11.
Levinas, E. (1982) *Difficile liberté*, Paris: Albin Michel.
Levine, P.M., Silberfarb, P.M., and Lipowski, Z.J. (1978) 'Mental disorders in cancer patients', *Cancer* 42: 1385–91.
Lévi-Strauss, C. (1966) *Mythologiques du miel aux cendres*, Paris: Plon.
Levy, S.M. (1985) *Behavior and cancer*, San Francisco: Jossey Bass.
Lewith, G.T. and Aldridge, D. (eds) (1993) *Clinical research methodology for complementary therapies*, London: Hodder & Stoughton.
Lichtenthaeler, C. (1978) *Histoire de la médecine*, Paris: Fayard.
Liebmann, M. (1986) *Art therapy for groups*, Beckenham: Croom Helm.
Linssen, A.C.G., Hanewald, J.G.F.P., Huisman, S., *et al.* (1982) 'The development of a well-being (quality of life) questionnaire at the Netherlands Cancer Institute', *Proceedings of the Third EORTC Workshop on Quality of Life*, Paris.
Lipowski, Z.J. (1970) 'Physical illness, the individual and the coping process', *Psychiatric Medicine* 1: 91–102.
Løfstrøm, B. (1969) 'Stellate ganglion block', in E. Eriksson (ed.) *Illustrated hand-book in local anesthesia*, Copenhagen: Sørensøn, 137–9.
Long, D.M. and Hagfors, N. (1975) 'Electrical stimulation of the nervous system: the current status of electrical stimulation of the nervous system for relief of pain', *Pain* 1: 109.
McCorkle, R. (1974) 'Effects of touch on seriously ill patients', *Nursing Research* 23: 125–32.
McGourty, H. (1993) *How to evaluate complementary therapies: a literature review*, Liverpool: Liverpool Public Health Observatory.
McIntosh, J. (1974) 'Process of communication, information seeking and control associated with cancer', *Social Science & Medicine* 8: 167–87.
McKechnie, A.A., Wilson, F., Watson, N., and Scott, D. (1983), 'Anxiety states: a preliminary report on the value of connective tissue massage', *Journal of Psychosomatic Research* 27: 125–9.
MacNutt, F. (1974) *Healing*, Notre Dame, Ind.: Ave Maria.
—— (1977) *The power to heal*, Notre Dame, Ind.: Ave Maria.
Magarey, C.J. (1981) 'Healing and meditation in medical practice', *Medical Journal of Australia* 338: 340–1.
—— (1983) 'Holistic cancer therapy', *Journal of Psychosomatic Research* 27 (3): 181–4.
Magarey, C.J., Todd, P.B., and Blizard, P.J. (1977) 'Psychosocial factors influencing delay and breast self-examination in women with symptoms of breast cancer', *Social Science & Medicine* 11: 229–39.
Maguire, G.P. (1984) 'The recognition and treatment of affective disorders in cancer patients', *International Review of Applied Psychology* 33: 479–81.

—— (1985) 'Improving the detection of psychiatric problems in cancer patients', *Social Science & Medicine* 20: 819–23.

Maguire, G.P., Brooke, M., Tait, A., *et al.* (1983) 'The effect of counselling on physical disability and social recovery after mastectomy', *Clinical Oncology* 9: 319–24.

Maguire, G.P., Lee, E.G., Bevington, D.J., *et al.* (1978) 'Psychiatric problems in the first year after mastectomy', *British Medical Journal* (i): 963–5.

Maillard, G.F., Pettavel, J., Viloux, D., *et al.* (1980) 'Aspects chirurgicaux et psychologiques de la reconstruction du sein après mastectomie', *Médecine & Hygiène* 38: 772.

Mandel, S. (1991) 'Music therapy in the hospice: "Musicalive"', *Palliative Medicine* 5: 155–60.

Mannoni, M. (1987) *Le divan de Procruste*, Paris: Denoël.

Marty, P. and M'Uzan, M. de, (1963) 'La pensée opératoire', *Revue Française de Psychanalyse* 27: 345–56.

Matthews Simonton, S. (1984) *The healing family*, New York: Bantam.

Meares, A. (1980) 'What can the cancer patient expect from intensive meditation?' *Australian Family Physician* 9: 322–5.

—— (1981) 'Regression of recurrence of carcinoma of the breast at mastectomy site associated with intensive meditation', *Australian Family Physician* 10: 218–9.

Mechanic, D. (1974) 'Social structure and personal adaptation: some neglected dimensions', in C.V. Ceolho, D.A. Hamburg, and J. Adams (eds) *Coping and adaptation*, New York: Basic Books, 32–44.

Melzack, R., Katz, J., and Jeans, M.E. (1985) 'The role of compensation in chronic pain: analysis using a new method of scoring the McGill Pain Questionnaire', *Pain* 23: 101–12.

Meyerowitz, B.E. (1980) 'Psychological correlates of breast cancer and its treatments', *Psychological Bulletin* 87: 108–31.

Meyerowitz, B.E., Sparks, F.C., and Spears, I.K. (1979) 'Adjuvant chemotherapy for breast carcinoma: psychosocial implications', *Cancer* 43: 1613–18.

Miller, C.L., Denner, P.R., and Richardson, V.E. (1976) 'Assisting the psychosocial problems of cancer patients: a review of current research', *International Journal of Nursing Studies* 13: 161–6.

Milton, G.W. (1973) 'Thoughts in mind of a person with cancer', *British Medical Journal* (iv): 221–3.

Minuchin, S. (1974) *Families and family therapy*, Cambridge, Mass.: Harvard University Press.

Moertel, C.G., Flemming, T.R., Rubin, J., *et al.* (1982) 'A clinical trial of amygdalin (laetrile) in the treatment of human cancer', *New England Journal of Medicine* 306: 201–6.

Mohl, P.C. (1980) 'A systems approach to liaison psychiatry', *Psychosomatics* 21: 457–61.

Monckton, J. (ed.) (1993) *The first ten years: 10th Anniversary Report 1983–1993*, London: Research Council for Complementary Medicine.

Moorey, S. and Greer, S. (1989) *Psychological therapy for patients with cancer: a new approach*, Oxford: Heinemann.

Morgan, W.L. and Engel, G.L. (1969) *The clinical approach to the patient*, Philadelphia: W.B. Saunders Co.

Morris, T. (1980) 'A "type" for cancer? Low trait anxiety in the pathogenesis of breast cancer', *Cancer Detection and Prevention* 3: 102.

Morris, T., Blake, S., and Buckley, M. (1985) 'Development of a method for rating cognitive responses to a diagnosis of cancer', *Social Science & Medicine* 20: 795–802.

Morris, T., Greer, S., and Keith, W. (1981) 'Patterns of expression of anger and their psychological correlates in women with breast cancer', *Journal of Psychosomatic Research* 25: 111–17.

Morris, T., Greer, H.S., and White, P. (1977) 'Psychological and social adjustment to mastectomy: a two-year follow-up study', *Cancer* 40: 2381–7.

Morrow, G.R. (1984) 'The assessment of nausea and vomiting: past problems, current issues, and suggestions for future research', *Cancer* 53: 2267–78.

Mosley, J.R. (1985) 'Alterations in comfort', *Nursing Clinics of North America* 20: 427–38.

Mount, B.M. (1980) *Vivre au jour le jour*, 16 mm film, Victoria Hospital, Montreal: Office national canadien du film.

Mount, B.M., Ajemian, I., and Scott, J.F. (1976) 'Use of the Brompton mixture in treating the chronic pain of malignant disease', *Canadian Medical Association Journal* 115: 122–4.

M'Uzan, M. de (1981) 'Dernières paroles', *Nouvelle Revue de Psychanalyse* 23: 117–30.

Nerenz, D.R., Leventhal, H., and Love, R.R. (1982) 'Factors contributing to emotional distress during cancer chemotherapy', *Cancer* 50: 1020–7.

Nou, E. and Aberg, T. (1980) 'Quality of survival in patients with surgically treated bronchial carcinoma', *Thorax* 35: 255–63.

Novack, D.H., Plumer, R., Smith, R.L., *et al.* (1979) 'Changes in physician's attitudes toward telling the cancer patient', *J A M A: The Journal of the American Medical Association* 241: 897–900.

Oken, D. (1961) 'What to tell cancer patients: a study of medical attitudes', *J A M A: The Journal of the American Medical Association* 175: 1120–8.

Palmer, S. and Bakshi, K. (1983) 'Diet, nutrition and cancer, interim dietary guidelines', *Journal of the National Cancer Institute* 70: 1151–70.

Pasini, W. and Andreoli, A. (1981) *Eros et changement – Le corps en psychothérapie*, Paris: Bibliothèque scientifique Payot.

Pattison, E.M. (1978) 'The living-dying process', in C.A. Garfield (ed.) *Psychosocial care of the dying patient*, New York: McGraw-Hill, 133–68.

Payne, R. and Foley, K.M. (1984) 'Advances in the management of cancer pain', *Cancer Treatment Reviews* 68: 173–83.

Pearlin, L.I. and Schooler, C. (1978) 'The structure of coping', *Journal of Health and Social Behavior* 19: 2–21.

Peteet, J.R. (1982) 'A closer look at the concept of support: some applications to the care of patients with cancer', *General Hospital Psychiatry* 4: 19–23.

Peters, G. (1981) 'Analgésie médicale', *Médecine & Hygiène* 40: 17–18.

Peters-Golden, H. (1982) 'Breast cancer: varied perceptions of social support in the illness experience', *Social Science & Medicine* 16: 483–91.

Pettingale, K.W., Greer, S., and Tee, D.E.H. (1977) 'Serum IgA and emotional expression in breast cancer patients', *Journal of Psychosomatic Research* 21: 395–9.

Pfefferbaum, B., Pasnau, R.O., Jamison, K., *et al.* (1977–8) 'A comprehensive program of psychosocial care for mastectomy patients', *International Journal of Psychiatry in Medicine* 8: 63.

Pierloot, R.A. (1983) 'Different models in the approach to the doctor–patient relationship', *Psychotherapy and Psychosomatics* 39: 213–24.

Pilowsky, I. and Spence, N.D. (1976) 'Pain, illness and behaviour: a comparative study', *Journal of Psychosomatic Research* 20: 131–4.

Plumb, M.M. and Holland, J. (1977) 'Comparative studies of psychological functions in patients with advanced cancer. I. Self-reported depressive symptoms', *Psychosomatic Medicine* 39: 264–76.

—— (1981) 'Comparative studies of psychological functions in patients with advanced cancer. III. Interviewer-rated current and past psychological symptoms', *Psychosomatic Medicine* 43: 243–54.

Poletti, R. (1984) 'La formation des infirmières à l'accompagnement du malade cancéreux', *Psychologie Médicale* 16: 2207–9.

Porter, J. and Jick, H. (1980) 'Addiction rare in patients treated with narcotics', *New England Journal of Medicine* 302: 123.

Priestman, T.J. and Baum, M. (1976) 'Evaluation of quality of life in patients receiving treatment of advanced breast cancer', *Lancet* (i): 899–901.

Priestman, T.J., Baum, M., and Priestman, S. (1981) 'The quality of life in breast cancer patients', in *Proceedings of the First EORTC Workshop on Quality of Life*, Amsterdam.

Pruyn, J.F.A., Rijckman, R.M., Brunschot, C.J.M. van, *et al.* (1985) 'Cancer patients' personality characteristics, physician–patient communication and adoption of the Moerman diet', *Social Science & Medicine* 20: 841–7.

Pullar, P. (1988) *Spiritual and lay healing*, Harmondsworth: Penguin.

Qureshi, B. (1989) *Transcultural medicine*, Lancaster: Kluwer.

Raimbault, E. (1984) 'Formation des spécialistes de psychologie médicale travaillant en cancérologie', *Psychologie Médicale* 16: 2203–5.

Reagan, T.J. and Okazaki, H. (1974) 'The thrombotic syndrome associated with carcinoma', *Archives of Neurology* 31: 390–5.

Redd, W.H. (1982) 'Behavioral analysis and control of psychosomatic symptoms of patients receiving intensive cancer treatment', *British Journal of Clinical Psychology* 21: 351–8.

Redd, W.H., Andresen, G.V., and Minagawa, R.Y. (1982a) 'Hypnotic control of anticipatory emesis in patients receiving cancer chemotherapy', *Journal of Consulting and Clinical Psychology* 50: 14–19.

Redd, W.H. and Andrykowski, M.A. (1982) 'Behavioral intervention in cancer treatment: controlling aversion reactions to chemotherapy', *Journal of Consulting and Clinical Psychology* 50: 1018–29.

Reik, T. (1948) *Listening with the third ear*, New York: Grove Press.

Renneker, R. (1981) 'Cancer and psychotherapy', in J.G. Goldberg (ed.) *Psychotherapeutic treatment of cancer patients*, New York: Free Press.

Reznikoff, M. (1955) 'Psychological factors in breast cancer', *Psychosomatic Medicine* 17: 96–108.

Reznikoff, M. and Martin, D. (1957) 'The influence of stress on mammary cancer', *Journal of Psychosomatic Research* 2: 56–8.

Richardson, P.H. and Vincent, C.A. (1986) 'Acupuncture for the treatment of pain: a review of evaluative research', *Pain* 24: 15–40.

Ringler, K.E., Whitman, H.H., Gustafson, J.P., *et al.* (1981) 'Technical advances in leading a cancer patient group', *International Journal of Group Psychotherapy* 31: 329–44.

Rosenthal, S. and Kaufman, S. (1974) 'Vincristine toxicity', *Annals of Internal Medicine* 80: 733–7.

Rusch, H.P. (1944) 'Extrinsic factors that influence carcinogenesis', *Physiological Reviews* 24: 177–204.

Sacerdote, P. (1966) 'The uses of hypnosis in cancer patients', *New York Academy of Sciences. Annals* 125: 1011–19.

Saks, M. (1992) *Alternative medicine in Britain*, Oxford: Oxford University Press.

Sapir, M. (1973) 'Médecine d'accompagnement', *Schweizerische Rundschau für Medizin Praxis* 62: 1473–6.

—— (1980) *Soignant-soigné: le corps à corps*, Paris: Payot.

—— (1984) 'La formation relationelle du généraliste face au patient cancéreux', *Psychologie Médicale* 16: 2191–3.

Saunders, D.C. (1982) 'Principles of symptom control in terminal care', *Medical Clinics of North America* 66: 1169–83.

Schafer, D.F. and Jones, E.A. (1982) 'Hepatic encephalopathy and the y-aminobutyric-acid neurotransmitter system', *Lancet* (i): 18–20.

Schain, W.S. (1982) 'Sexual problems of patients with cancer', in V.T. DeVita, S. Hellman, and S.A. Rosenberg (eds) *Cancer: principles and practice of oncology*, Philadelphia: J.B. Lippincott, 278–91.

Scheder, P.A. (1986) 'Médecines alternatives et orientation vers la prévention de leurs usagers', *Médecine & Hygiène* 44: 384–90.

Schilsky, R.L., Lewis, B.J., Sherins, R.J., *et al.* (1980) 'Gonadal dysfunction in patients receiving chemotherapy for cancer', *Annals of Internal Medicine* 93: 109–14.

Schmale, A.H., Jr (1984) 'Response to Wortman', *Cancer* 53: 2360–2.

Schmale, A.H., Jr and Iker, H.P. (1964) 'The effect of hopelessness in the development of cancer. Part I: The prediction of uterine cervical cancer in women with atypical cytology', *Psychosomatic Medicine* 26: 634–5.

—— (1966) 'The psychological setting of uterine cervical cancer', *New York Academy of Sciences. Annals* 125: 807–13.

Schneider, P.-B. (1969a) *Psychologie Médicale*, Paris: Payot.

—— (1969b) 'Médecine psychosomatique, mythe ou réalité?', *Gynecologica* 167: 69–80.

—— (1976) *Propédeutique d'une psychothérapie*, Paris: Payot, 49–69.

—— (1978) 'La psychologie médicale; Pourquoi? Comment?', *La vie médicale au Canada français* 7: 491–502.

—— (1980) 'Le médecin: l'inconnu de la psychologie médicale', *Psychologie Médicale* 12: 1233–43.

—— (1985) 'Formation Balint et aspects psychothérapiques: introduction', *Psychologie Médicale* 17: 2059–66.

Schnorrenberger, C.C. (1979) 'Thérapeutique chinoise traditionelle',

Bulletin Sandoz 51: 15–22.

Schonfield, J. (1972) 'Psychological factors related to delayed return to an earlier life-style in successfully treated cancer patients', *Journal of Psychosomatic Research* 16: 41–6.

—— (1975) 'Psychological and life experience differences between Israeli women with benign and cancerous breast lesions', *Journal of Psychosomatic Research* 19: 229–34.

Schraub, S., Gauley-Mosdier, M.C., and Bosset, J.F. (1982) 'Les thérapeutiques parallèles du cancer', *Médecine & Hygiène* 40: 1415–26.

Schulz, R. and Aderman, D. (1974) 'Clinical research and the stages of dying', *Omega* 5: 137–43.

Segaloff, A. (1981) 'Managing endocrine metabolic problems in the patient with advanced cancer', *J A M A: The Journal of the American Medical Association* 245: 177–9.

Seigel, L.J. and Longon, D.L. (1981) 'The control of chemotherapy-induced emesis', *Annals of Internal Medicine* 95: 352–9.

Sewell, H.H. and Edwards, D.W. (1980) 'Pelvic genital cancer: body image and sexuality', *Frontiers of Radiation Therapy and Oncology* 14: 35–41.

Sharma, U. (1992) *Complementary medicine today*, London: Routledge.

Shekelle, R.B., Raynor, W.J., Ostfeld, A.M., et al. (1981) 'Psychological depression and 17-year risk of death from cancer', *Psychosomatic Medicine* 43: 117–25.

Siegrist, J.F. (1976) 'Asymmetrische Kommunikation bei klinischen Visiten', *Medizinische Klinik* 45: 1962–6.

Silberfarb, P.M. (1984a) 'Psychiatric problems in breast cancer', *Cancer* 53: 820–4.

—— (1984b) 'Response to Folstein', *Cancer* 53: 2255–7.

Silberfarb, P.M., Holland, J.C.B., Anbar, D., et al. (1983) 'Psychological response of patients receiving two drug regimens for lung carcinoma', *American Journal of Psychiatry* 140: 110–11.

Silberfarb, P.M., Maurer, L.H., and Crouthamel, C.S. (1980a) 'Psychosocial aspects of neoplastic disease. I: Functional status of breast cancer patients during different treatment regimens', *American Journal of Psychiatry* 137: 450–5.

Silberfarb, P.M., Philibert, D., and Levine, P.M. (1980b) 'Psychosocial aspects of neoplastic disease. II: Affective and cognitive effects of chemotherapy in cancer patients', *American Journal of Psychiatry* 137: 597–601.

Silver, R.L. and Wortman, C.B. (1980) 'Coping with undesirable life events', in J. Garber and M.E.P. Seligman (eds) *Human helplessness: theory and applications*, New York: Academic Press, 279–345.

Simonton, O.C., Matthews Simonton, S., and Creighton, J.L. (1978) *Getting well again*, New York: J.P. Tarcher.

Singer, J.E. (1984) 'Some issues in the study of coping', *Cancer* 53: 2303–13.

Sklar, L.S. and Anisman, H. (1980) 'Social stress influences tumor growth', *Psychosomatic Medicine* 42: 347–65.

Soni, S.S., Marten, G.W., Pitner, S.E., et al. (1975) 'Effects of central-nervous-system irradiation on neuropsychologic functioning of children with acute lymphocytic leukemia', *New England Journal of Medicine* 293: 113–18.

Spence, K.W. (1964) 'Anxiety (drive) level and performance in eyelid conditioning', *Psychological Bulletin* 61: 129–39.

Spiegel, D. and Bloom, J.R. (1983) 'Pain in metastatic breast cancer', *Cancer* 52: 341–5.

Spiegel, D., Bloom, J.R., Kraemer, H.C., and Gottheil, E. (1989) 'Effect of psychosocial treatment on survival of patients with metastatic breast cancer', *Lancet* (ii): 888–91.

Spiegel, D., Bloom, J.R., and Yalom, I. (1981) 'Group support for patients with metastatic cancer', *Archives of General Psychiatry* 38: 527–33.

Spielberger, C.D. (1975) 'Anxiety: state-trait process', in C.D. Spielberger and I.G. Sarason (eds) *Stress and anxiety*, vol. 2, Washington, D.C.: Hemisphere, 115–43.

Staps, T., Hoogenhout, J., and Wobbes, T. (1985) 'Phantom breast sensations following mastectomy', *Cancer* 56: 2898.

Sternbach, R.A. (1974) *Pain patients: traits and treatment*, New York: Academic Press.

Stevens, C. (1987) *Alexander technique*, London: Macdonald.

Stevens, L.A., McGrath, M.H., Druss, R.G., *et al.* (1984) 'The psychological impact of immediate breast reconstruction for women with early breast cancer', *Plastic and Reconstructive Surgery* 73: 619.

Stiefel, F.C., Breitbart, W.S., and Holland, J.C. (1989) 'Corticosteroids in cancer: neuropsychiatric complications', *Cancer Investigation* 7 (5): 479–91.

Storr, A. (1992) *Music and the mind*, London: Harper Collins.

Stoudemire, A., Cotanch, P., and Laszlo, J. (1984) 'Recent advances in the pharmacologic and behavioral management of chemotherapy-induced emesis', *Archives of Internal Medicine* 144: 1029–33.

Sugerbaker, P.H., Barofsky, I., Rosenberg, S.A., *et al.* (1982) 'Quality of life assessment of patients in extremity sarcoma clinical trials', *Surgery* 91: 17–23.

Tarnower, W. (1984) 'Psychotherapy with cancer patients', *Bulletin of the Menninger Clinic* 48: 342–50.

Temoshok, L. (1985) 'Biopsychosocial studies on cutaneous melanoma: psychosocial factors associated with prognostic indicators, progression, psychophysiology and tumor-host response', *Social Science & Medicine* 20: 833–40.

Thachil, J.V., Jewett, M.A.S., and Rider, W.D. (1981) 'The effects of cancer and therapy on male fertility', *Journal of Urology* 126: 141–5.

Theologides, A. (1972) 'Pathogenesis of cachexia in cancer', *Cancer* 29: 484–8.

Thomas, C.B. and Duszynski, K.R. (1974) 'Closeness to parents and the family constellation in a prospective study of five disease states: suicide, mental illness, malignant tumor, hypertension and coronary heart disease', *Hopkins Medical Journal* 134: 251–70.

Thomas, C.B. and Greenstreet, R.L. (1973) 'Psychobiological character-istics in youth as predictors of five disease states: suicide, mental illness, hypertension, coronary heart disease and tumor', *Hopkins Medical Journal* 16: 132–44.

Thomas, P.R.M., Winstanly, D., Peckham, M.J., *et al.* (1976) 'Reproductive

and endocrine function in patients with Hodgkin's disease: effects of
oophoropexy and irradiation', *British Journal of Cancer* 33: 226–31.

Thomson, R. (1989) *Loving medicine: patients' experiences of the Bristol Cancer Help Centre*, Bath: Gateway.

Tilliette, X. (1985) 'Mourir, survivre?', *Etudes* 363: 91–104.

Tune, L.E., Holland, A., Folstein, M.F., *et al.* (1981) 'Association of postoperative delirium with raised serum levels of anticholinergic drugs', *Lancet* (ii): 651–2.

Turner, J.A. and Chapman, C.R. (1982) 'Psychological interventions for chronic pain: a critical review. II: Operant conditioning hypnosis and cognitive-behavioral therapy', *Pain* 12: 23–46.

Twentyman, R. (1989) *The science and art of healing*, Edinburgh: Floris Books.

Twycross, R.G. and Fairfield, S. (1982) 'Pain in far-advanced cancer', *Pain* 14: 303–10.

Twycross, R.G. and Lack, S.A. (1984) *Symptom control in far-advanced cancer: Pain relief*, London: Pitman.

Tyner, R. (1985) 'Elements of empathic care for dying patients and their families', *Nursing Clinics of North America* 20: 393–401.

Vaillant, G.E. (1977) *Adaptation to life*, Boston: Little Brown.

Vayer, P. (1973) *Le dialogue corporel*, Paris: Doin.

Vera, M.I. (1981) 'Quality of life following pelvic exenteration', *Gynecologic Oncology* 12: 355–66.

Verwoerdt, A. (1966) *Communication with the fatally ill*, Springfield, Ill.: C.C. Thomas.

Vincent, C.E., Vincent, B., Greiss, R.C., *et al.* (1975) 'Some marital-sexual concomitants of carcinoma of cervix', *Southern Medical Journal* 68: 552–8.

Vissing, Y.M. and Petersen, J.C. (1981) 'Taking laetrile: conversion to medical deviance', *Ca – A Cancer Journal for Clinicians* 31: 365–9.

Walshe, W.H. (1846) *The nature and treatment of cancer*, London: Taylor & Walton.

Ward, N.G., Bloom, V.L., and Friedel, R.O. (1979) 'The effectiveness of tricyclic antidepressants in the treatment of coexisting pain and depression', *Pain* 7: 331–41.

Watson, M. and Greer, S. (1983) 'Development of a questionnaire measure of emotional control', *Journal of Psychosomatic Research* 27: 299–305.

Webb, W.L. and Gehl, M. (1981) 'Electrolyte and fluid imbalance: neuropsychiatric manifestations', *Psychosomatics* 22: 199–203.

Weddington, W.W. (1982) 'Psychogenic nausea and vomiting associated with termination of cancer chemotherapy', *Psychotherapy and Psychosomatics* 37: 129–36.

Weeks, N. (1940) *The medical discoveries of Edward Bach, physician*, Saffron Walden: C.W. Daniel.

Weisman, A. (1976) 'Coping behavior and suicide in cancer', in J.W. Cullen, B.H. Fox, and R.N. Isom (eds) *Cancer: the behavioral dimensions*, New York: Raven Press.

Weisman, A.D. and Sobel, H.J. (1979) 'Coping with cancer through self-instruction: a hypothesis', *Journal of Human Stress*, 3–8.

Weisman, A. and Worden, J. (1975) 'Psychosocial analysis of cancer deaths', *Omega* 6: 61–75.

—— (1976–7) 'The existential plight in cancer: significance of the first 100 days', *International Journal of Psychiatry in Medicine* 7(1): 1–15.

Welch, D.A. (1980) 'Assessment of nausea and vomiting in cancer patients undergoing external beam radiotherapy', *Cancer Nursing* 3: 365–71.

Wellisch, D.K. (1979) 'Adolescent acting out when a parent has cancer', *International Journal of Family Therapy* 1: 230–41.

—— (1984) 'Work, social, recreation, family and physical status', *Cancer* 53: 2290–9.

Wellisch, D.K., Schain, W.S., Barrett Noone, R., *et al.* (1985) 'Psychosocial correlates of immediate versus delayed reconstruction of the breast', *Plastic and Reconstructive Surgery* 76: 713.

Wenjun, Y. (1988) 'Investigation into a new system for the treatment of cancer with Chinese medicinal substances', *Journal of Chinese Medicine* 26: 29–35.

Whitehead, V.M. (1975) 'Cancer treatment needs better antiemetics', *New England Journal of Medicine* 293: 199–200.

Williams, P.A. (1983) 'Cancer and the family physician', *Cancer* 52: 2410–12.

Wirsching, M., Stierlin, H., Haas, B., *et al.* (1981) 'Familientherapie bei Krebsleiden', *Familiendynamik* 6: 1–23.

Wirsching, M., Stierlin, H., Hoffman, F., *et al.* (1982) 'Psychological identification of breast cancer patients before biopsy', *Journal of Psychosomatic Research* 26: 1–10.

Wise, T.N. (1979) 'Sexuality in chronic illness', *Primary Care* 4: 199–208.

Worden, J. and Weisman, A. (1980) 'Do cancer patients really want counseling?', *General Hospital Psychiatry* 2: 100–3.

Wortman, C. and Dunkel-Schetter, C. (1979) 'Interpersonal relationships and cancer: a theoretical analysis', *Journal of Social Issues* 35: 120–55.

Wortman, C.B. (1984) 'Social support and the cancer patient. Conceptual and methodologic issues', *Cancer* 53: 2339–60.

Zack, M.V. (1985) 'Loneliness: a concept relevant to the care of dying persons', *Nursing Clinics of North America* 20: 403–13.

Zigmond, A.S. and Snaith, R.P. (1983) 'The Hospital Anxiety and Depression Scale', *Acta Psychiatrica Scandinavica* 67: 361–70.

Zumbrunnen, R. (1992) *Psychiatrie de liaison*, Paris: Masson.

Some useful organizations

American Cancer Society
1599 Clifton Road N.E., Atlanta, Georgia 30329, USA
Tel. (404) 320 3333   Fax (404) 325 0230

Nationwide community-based voluntary health organization
dedicated to preventing cancer, saving lives from cancer, and
diminishing suffering from cancer through research, education,
and service to patients and families. Operates a cancer information
hotline, organizes conferences and publishes newsletters and
journals such as *World, Smoking & Health* and *Ca – A Cancer
Journal for Clinicians.*

American Society of Psychiatric Oncology/AIDS
President: Mary Jane Massie, M.D.
1275 York Avenue, Box 421, New York, NY 10021, USA
Tel. (212) 639 8010   Fax (212) 717 3087

Established in 1988, ASPOA serves as a network to exchange
information about psychiatric and psychobiological aspects of
oncology and AIDS and to foster research and training. The
clinical goal is to promote the psychosocial, psychiatric,
behavioural and ethical aspects of care for patients with cancer
and AIDS. Scientific meetings are held biannually and members
receive the journal *Psycho-Oncology.*

ASPECT (registered as The Jeannie Campbell Breast Cancer
Radiotherapy Appeal)
29 St Luke's Avenue, Ramsgate, Kent CT11 7JZ, UK
Tel. 0843 596732   Fax 0843 853184

A small charity specializing in help for breast cancer patients. Publishes a set of free leaflets, especially on hormonal treatments (Tamoxifen, Megace), for patients and health professionals.

Australian Association for Hospice and Palliative Care
P.O. Box 1200, North Fitzroy, Victoria 3068, Australia
Tel. (03) 486 2666   Fax (03) 482 5094

With its member State Associations, promotes and advocates the principles of palliative care, and the equitable development of hospice and palliative care services for persons with a terminal illness and their families throughout Australia.

Australian Cancer Society Inc.
153 Dowling Street, Woolloomooloo, NSW 2011, Australia
Tel. (02) 358 2066   Fax (02) 356 4558

The national office for the State and Territory cancer organizations responsible in their own regions for funding research, professional and public education, and counselling and support services for cancer patients and families. Publishes *Cancer Forum*, and is the link with Government and overseas cancer organizations.

Breast Care and Mastectomy Association (BCMA)
15–19 Britten Street, London SW3 3TZ, UK
Tel. 071 867 1103 (helpline); 071 867 8275 (administration); 041 353 1050 (Glasgow helpline)

A national organization offering free help, information and support to women with breast cancer. There is a prosthesis advisory service and a network of trained volunteers with personal experience of breast surgery who offer one-to-one emotional support. Information available for health professionals.

Bristol Cancer Help Centre
Grove House, Cornwallis Grove, Clifton, Bristol BS8 4PG, UK
Tel. 0272 743216   Fax 0272 239184

One-day and one-week holistic courses (led by doctors) for cancer patients which include counselling, relaxation, visualization, meditation, art and music therapy, healing, and dietary advice. Seminars and courses for health professionals.

British Association for Cancer United Patients (BACUP)
3 Bath Place, Rivington Street, London EC2A 3JR, UK
Tel. 071 613 2121 (London callers); 0800 181199 (free helpline outside London); 071 696 9003 (administration); 071 696 9000 (counselling)

Cancer nurses provide free, confidential information and emotional support to patients, relatives and friends. The London-based counselling service offers up to eight free sessions. Over 40 publications on various cancers. A resource for health professionals as well as patients.

British Association for Counselling
1 Regent Place, Rugby, Warwickshire, CV21 2PJ, UK
Tel. 0788 578328 (information); 0788 550899 (administration)

Publishes the quarterly journal *Counselling*, has developed a Code of Ethics and Practice for counsellors and an accreditation scheme, and publishes directories describing training and counselling services. The 'Counselling in Medical Settings' Division publishes a quarterly journal, *CMS News*.

British Holistic Medical Association
179 Gloucester Place, London NW1 6DX, UK
Tel. 071 262 5299

An association for health professionals and others who want to adopt a more holistic approach in their own life and work, and to re-integrate psychological and spiritual dimensions into health care. Publishes a quarterly newsletter, *Holistic Health*.

British Psychosocial Oncology Group (BPOG)
Membership Secretary: Judy Young
Cancer Support and Information Centre, Mount Vernon Hospital
Northwood, Middlesex, HA6 2RN, UK
Tel. 0895 278177 (Cancer support helpline 0895 278014)

A professional association formed to encourage communication between different professional groups interested in the psychological and social factors associated with cancer. Publishes a twice-yearly newsletter and the quarterly journal *Psycho-Oncology*. An annual conference with international speakers is organized where developments in the field can be reviewed and new research findings presented. Supports occasional workshops on special topics.

Canadian Cancer Society

10 Alcorn Avenue, Suite 200, Toronto, Ontario M4V 3B1, Canada
Tel. (416) 961 7223   Fax (416) 961 4189

A national community-based organization of volunteers. The
Society believes that emotional and psychological support is as
important as medical treatment to the quality of life of people
living with cancer. Volunteers, many of whom have had a personal
experience with cancer, are available to meet with patients and
their families to offer emotional support. Both one-to-one visits
and group discussions are available.

Cancer Relief Macmillan Fund

15–19 Britten Street, London SW3 3TZ, UK
Tel. 071 351 7811

A national charity aiming to improve the lives of people with
cancer at any stage of the disease and in any setting – whether at
home, in hospital, or in a specialized cancer unit. Macmillan
nurses are trained in counselling, and in pain and symptom
control. CRMF provides financial support to cancer patients, and
also funds a medical support and education programme to improve
the skills of doctors and nurses in cancer care.

Cancer Society of NZ Incorporated

PO Box 12145, Wellington, New Zealand
Tel. (04) 473 6409   Fax (04) 499 0849

A voluntary organization comprising six autonomous regional
Divisions providing support services for cancer patients and their
families, research funding, health promotion and professional
education.

CancerLink

17 Britannia Street, London WC1X 9JN, UK
Tel. and textphone (use voice announcer) 071 833 2451
(information service); 071 833 2818 (groups and individual
supporters); 071 713 7867 (Asian language line: Hindi, Bengali);
031 228 5557 (Edinburgh helpline). Free 'Mac' helpline for young
people 0800 591028

Provides emotional support and information in response to
telephone and letter enquiries on all aspects of cancer, from people

with cancer, their families and friends, and from professionals working with them. Gives assistance and training to over 450 cancer self-help and support groups throughout the UK, issues a wide range of publications including a directory of support groups (with an international section), and helps people who set up new groups.

Carers National Association
20–25 Glasshouse Yard, London EC1A 4JS, UK
Tel. 071 490 8818

Provides support and information to people caring for relatives at home. There is a national network of local branches and offices.

Clinical Oncological Society of Australia Inc.
153 Dowling Street, Woolloomooloo, NSW 2011, Australia
Tel. (02) 358 2066   Fax (02) 356 4558

A special medical society for clinicians, scientists, and allied health professionals, including oncological nurses and social workers, formed for the exchange and dissemination of information on research, clinical practice, and patient care. Includes a psycho-oncology sub-group.

CRUSE
Cruse House, 126 Sheen Road, Richmond, Surrey TW9 1UR, UK
Tel. 081 940 4818 (information); 081 332 7227 (direct link to a counsellor)

A national organization offering a counselling service for the bereaved, staffed by trained volunteers.

Hospice Information Service
St Christopher's Hospice, 51–59 Lawrie Park Road, Sydenham, London SE26 6DZ, UK
Tel. 081 778 9252

A resource for members of the public and health-care professionals seeking information on the work of the hospice movement in the UK and overseas. A worldwide *Directory of Hospice Services* is available.

Institute for Complementary Medicine
PO Box 194, London SE16 1QZ, UK
Tel. 071 237 5165

Supplies names of registered practitioners of various kinds of
complementary medicine. Send s.a.e. for information, stating area
of interest.

International Federation of Medical Psychology Organizations
General Secretary: Professor Patrice Guex
Division de Médecine Psycho-Sociale, BH 07
CHUV, 1011 Lausanne, Switzerland
Tel. (021) 314 40 51   Fax (021) 314 40 56

Founded in 1975, the Federation aims to stimulate research,
information, teaching and training in the fields of medical
psychology, psychosomatic medicine, medical psycho-sociology,
and in general, human science applied to medicine. Runs
international conferences and seminars.

International Psycho-Oncology Society
Executive Secretary: Anthony Marchini, M.S.
Memorial Sloan-Kettering Cancer Center
1275 York Avenue, Box 421, New York, NY 10021, USA
Tel. (212) 639 7051   Fax (212) 717 3087

Fosters international multidisciplinary communication about
clinical, educational and research issues related to the
psychosocial dimensions of cancer: the response of patients,
families and staff to cancer and its treatment at all stages, and the
psychological, social, and behavioural factors that influence
tumour progression and survival. Seeks to develop standards in
educational training and research in these areas. Conducts/co-
sponsors international meetings.

Irish Cancer Society
5 Northumberland Road, Dublin 4, Republic of Ireland
Tel. (01) 6681855 (administration); (01) 6681233 (helpline)

The helpline service offers information on all aspects of cancer.
The society also funds home care and rehabilitation for cancer
patients, and runs support groups for mastectomy, colostomy,
laryngectomy, and other patients.

Leeds Medical Information

University of Leeds, Leeds LS2 9JT, UK
Tel. 0532 335550   Fax 0532 334381

Publishes the bi-monthly journals *Progress in Palliative Care* and *Current Clinical Cancer*, a monthly index of the international journal literature of clinical oncology, both of which include material on psychosocial oncology, and also a series of current awareness titles on cancer virology and AIDS and HIV infection.

Marie Curie Cancer Care

28 Belgrave Square, London SW1X 8QG, UK
Tel. 071 235 3325

A charity that provides nursing care and hospices for cancer patients. It also runs training courses for health professionals in cancer care and prevention.

National Cancer Institute

Building 31, Room 10A24, 9000 Rockville Pike, Bethesda, Maryland 20892, USA
Tel. (301) 496 5583   Fax (301) 402 2594

The NCI co-ordinates national cancer research. It has built a network of cancer centres, cancer physicians, co-operative groups of clinical researchers, volunteer and community outreach groups, and state and local health departments. The Cancer Information Service (toll free 1–800–4–CANCER) answers cancer-related questions from the public, cancer patients and their families, and health professionals.

Oncology Nursing Society

501 Holiday Drive, Pittsburgh, PA 15220–2749, USA
Tel. (412) 921 7373   Fax (412) 921 6565

The ONS is a national organization of more than 24,000 registered nurses dedicated to excellence in patient care, teaching, research and education in the field of oncology. Publishes the *Oncology Nursing Forum* and offers a variety of educational conferences.

PLUS Self Help Association

Cramond House, Kirk Cramond, Cramond Glebe Road, Edinburgh EH4 6NS, UK
Tel. 031 312 7955

PLUS stands for 'Positive Living Under Stress'. It aims to establish new support groups for people with cancer, carers and the bereaved, throughout Scotland. The national office offers information and support to new and existing groups, and training in counselling and support skills.

Research Council for Complementary Medicine
60 Great Ormond Street, London WC1N 3JF, UK
Tel. 071 833 8897   Fax 071 278 7412

Fosters, enables, and sponsors research into the complementary therapies and promotes greater distribution of information on research results in order to bring about wider options in health care.

Tak Tent Cancer Support Scotland
G Block, 4th floor, Western Infirmary, Dumbarton Road, Glasgow G11 6NT, UK
Tel. 041 334 6699

Offers emotional support and information on cancers and treatments for patients, relatives, and professionals. There are support groups throughout Scotland.

Tenovus Cancer Information Centre
142 Whitchurch Road, Cardiff, South Glamorgan CF4 3NA, UK
Tel. 0222 619846 (administration); 0800 526527 (free helpline)

Information and advice about cancer and its prevention. The helpline is staffed by trained nurses, counsellors, and social workers.

Ulster Cancer Foundation
40–42 Eglantine Avenue, Belfast BT9 6DX, UK
Tel. 0232 663281 (administration); 0232 663439 (helpline)

The helpline, staffed by cancer nurses, offers information and support for patients and their families. Personal counselling is also available at the centre.

Appendix 2

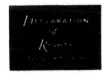

This Declaration of Rights of People with Cancer has been produced by CancerLink to bring the needs of people with cancer to the attention of health professionals, employers and the public at large.

The document is designed to act as a starting point for debate about how the needs of people with cancer are being met and how service provision could be improved.

The following do not all exist as legal rights but are felt to be fundamental to the well being of people with cancer.

I have the right:

1. ... to equal concern and attention whatever my gender, race, class, culture, religious belief, age, sexuality, lifestyle, or degree of able-bodiedness.

2. ... to be considered with respect and dignity, and to have my physical, emotional, spiritual, social and psychological needs taken seriously and responded to throughout my life, whatever my prognosis.

3. ... to know I have cancer, to be told in a sensitive manner and to share in all decision-making about my treatment and care in honest and informative discussions with relevant specialists and other health professionals.

4. ... to be informed fully about treatment options and to have explained to me the benefits, side effects and risks of any treatment.

5. ... to be asked for my informed consent before I am entered into any clinical trial.

6. ... to a second opinion, to refuse treatment or to use complementary therapies without prejudice to continued medical support.

7. ... to have any special welfare needs acknowledged and benefit claims responded to promptly.

8. ... to be employed, promoted or accepted on return to work according to my abilities and experience and not according to assumptions about my disease and its progression.

9. ... to easy access to information about local and national services, cancer support and self help groups and practitioners that may be useful in meeting my needs.

10. ... to receive support and information to help me understand and come to terms with my disease, and to receive similar support for my family and friends.

This declaration is reproduced by kind permission of the British national charity CancerLink, who published and launched it in September 1990

Index

Milton Keynes UK
Ingram Content Group UK Ltd.
UKHW040013071024
449327UK00011B/202